WHEN THE WHEELS
OF FAITH QUIT TURNING

A Book About Breast Cancer

A Book of Love, Faith, Unity and Strength

By

Earlene Jernigan-Carter

Earlene Jernigan-Carter
jerniganearlene@yahoo.com

First Printing 1996

Revised 2009

Manufactured in the United States of America

Bible Quotes from The Holy Bible
The King James Version

Cover Photo by Lester Carter Jr.

ISBN 978-0-557-17231-3

WHEN THE WHEELS
OF FAITH QUIT TURNING

"We then that are strong ought to bear the infirmities of the weak, and not to please ourselves."

Romans 15:1

FOREWORD AND DEDICATION

My personal story reveals some difficult moments that might have measured intolerable had there not been some very patient and competent people there to help me. This story examines my feelings before and after others reached out to me. It communicates the manner in which I adapted, once I was encouraged to accept change. It is about God's gifts of love, faith, unity and strength that prevailed during my illness, throughout my chemotherapy treatments, and on into recovery.

It is my hope that this book will be informative and resound a message of thanks to all who were so kind and obedient to God's will for my sake.

To Dr. Bodden, Dr. Fosmire, Dr. Knox, Dr. Jones, Dr. Porter, Dr. Sones, the staff at the Dallas Medical and Surgical Clinic, The Oncology Center, Baylor Medical Hospital and it's affiliates, I thank God for your professional gifts in the medical field. Thank you for exercising those gifts with competence, expedience, and patience.

To my family, Dr. Knox, Jerry and Thelma Darden, Dessie Minor, Lawrence and Doris and Justin Giles, Pastor A.C. Toney and other members of the Pleasant Zion Missionary Baptist Church, Orr Hinton, Charolyn Sifford, and other co-workers in the Public Works Department.

And I will remember—for the rest of my life—the conversations with Aunt Betty and Henrietta and the hospital's support staff that got me through the really tough chemotherapy sessions. Their first hand experiences of chemotherapy, shared through those conversations, were testimonies that God knows just how much we can really bear.

For seeing that I always had an appropriate meal at home—to Aunt Betty, sister-in-law Ruby, and co-workers—thank you.

And even beyond that—for seeing that I had other necessities and help with housework if I needed—many thanks to a good friend and co-worker, Modesta Pena.

For seeing that my benefits were properly addressed, I am grateful to Wonder Joe and Linda Gleghorn in Public Works Administration, along with my department manager, Barbara Reading and Bhgwan Shaw (who kept up with my time).

To my sister Lois, my sister-in-law Ruby, Lester Sr., co-workers Tom Berry, Orr Hinton, Jerry Darden and Bhgwan Shaw, thank you for transportation whenever I needed to go for doctor's appointments. For those days when I was sick at work and needed to go home, many thanks also to Elaine Hubbard and Kathy McCullough for taking me home.

I thank all of my family—my sister Lois here in Dallas (who sat by my bed many hours and communicated progress reports to the family); my mother (whose overwhelming concern caused her to be hospitalized during this awesome time), my sister Clarine and my brothers, Eddie and wife Eloise, Alvin and J.D. (miles away) who prayed and called—who sent me flowers and cards. Thank you for remembering and caring that my children and I still needed you even though friends were around. Thank you for accepting with me their gifts of love.

To my children, Marfa and Lester, Jr., thank you for all your help and for trying to understand. This book is especially dedicated to you.

To families who have lost love ones to cancer, and others who are still suffering, I pray that God will give you comfort and peace. To those who continue the search for a cure, I thank God for your perseverance. This book is also dedicated to all of you.

Conclusively, this book would not be complete without special thanks to my daughter and to one of my closest friends, Glenn Tolbert for the use of their typewriters on my first draft. For the cover of this book, I am grateful to my son Lester Jr. who provided me with the cover photo. For proofing portions of my manuscript and encouraging me to continuing my writing, in pursuit of my dreams for publication of this story, the list is endless. I thank you all for continuously asking, "Where's the book?"

May God richly bless you all!

INTRODUCTION

When I learned that I had breast cancer, I was a single parent with two teen-age children; a nineteen year old daughter who had just graduated from high school and a son who was turning thirteen. The three of us shared mixed feelings of fear, anger, insecurity and sometimes guilt for not being there for each other regardless of the circumstances. This disease caught us off guard and tampered with our goals and focal points on a daily basis, and we all had to learn a kind of independence on our own that we had only seen at a distance in the lives of others. Then after the surgery, the physical and emotional pain seemed almost unbearable for me and caused life changing moments.

However, with time, encouragement, and constant reminders from family and friends, we shared a much deeper meaning for life. The end result has been strength and faith to endure bigger challenges. I experienced and maintain, to this day, a closer bond with God.

In this revised addition, there are several corrections and some expanded reading. If you have purchased a copy of this book or the one before, I thank you. We can all make a difference for those diagnosed with this dreadful disease by extending a helping hand to their extended needs. May God bless that the journey will not be in vain.

CONTENTS

WHEN THE WHEELS
OF FAITH QUIT TURNING

Chapter 1

Should I Get My Coat Lord

Reminiscing for a moment of hope or in search of my faith, I felt betrayed by the old cliché that at age forty I would be enjoying the best of the rest of my life. Only now, I wondered if it was too late to look back on the rest of that cliché, "If you take care of yourself."

It was like the wheels of faith just quit turning. There had been signals to slow me down and to make me pay attention, but I kept putting it off to get myself checked out.

I had turned too late as I approached the corner of my living room wall, and I accidentally bumped my right breast. It was throbbing like a mild headache. I didn't think anything was seriously wrong until I noticed that my breast was getting sore and swelling. Even then, I didn't go to the doctor right away.

And—how could I have forgotten that just a little over a year had gone by since I was in Baylor Hospital's emergency room; the end result, removal of fibroid tumors from my uterine wall. Dr. Lux performed that surgery at Baylor since I had not been able to get an appointment sooner at the Dallas Medical and Surgical Clinic.

Over ten years prior, Dr. Fosmire had performed surgery at the Dallas Medical and Surgical Clinic to remove benign cyst from both breast. Each time I had been reminded that I should come in for regular checkups.

Unfortunately, my doctor had left the clinic, and I hesitated to make an appointment to see another doctor until my symptoms continued. Several months went by. It was time for my physical anyway, and since the knot felt bigger, I decided that I'd better go get a checkup this time. The knot felt to be half the size of a jack ball.

Thursday, February 7, 1991, I made an appointment at the Clinic to see the Gynecologist, Dr. Vernie Bodden. After examining me, Dr. Bodden sent me up to see the Surgeon, Dr. Fosmire.

Dr. Fosmire examined me and sent me up to the lab for x-rays and a mammography. I knew something very serious was wrong by the way the technician responded. I don't recall what she said, except I do remember one of the nurses asking, "Whose file is this? Bless her heart."

They didn't give me the file. I guessed they didn't want me to learn of the result before Dr. Fosmire had a chance to talk to me. Besides, he always told me things himself directly. So I went back to Dr. Fosmire's office and the nurse brought him the file with the x-rays. That's when he sat down with me to discuss everything.

As I expected, Dr. Fosmire recommended that I come into the hospital to get the knot removed. Only it wasn't just a knot. Now I would come to know a different set of meaningful words as Dr. Fosmire spoke: tumor, cancer, operation, and mastectomy. I understood all but one word—mastectomy—and after he explained, I wished for another word.

Ironically, my heart seemed so heavy that I was no longer sitting up straight, causing my back to hurt. To further intensify the situation, the throbbing pain from the knot, that I had paid little attention to before, was more noticeable also. No matter what Dr. Fosmire said, I was entertaining a million questions and thoughts of my own.

"Oh my God no!" How could this have just happened? Will I get infected and die on the operating table? Have I waited too late? Are the doctors really giving me the only alternative to this situation?"

I wanted to promise God everything that I could. Only there was nothing more precious to me than my own life, and he already had total control of that.

As Dr. Fosmire continued to talk to me about operating, I thanked God that there was still hope. I felt grateful for my health being as well as it was—especially looking back on my life.

Besides my consumption of what was obviously contributing to ill will, nature had long before notified me of my imperfect health. During my childhood, I had constant nosebleeds (from the summer heat, dust or other unknown causes) whooping cough and measles simultaneously, and an eye operation before I was seven years old. Not long after that, I had spinal meningitis that left me with a weak back. As I got older, I experienced cramps so bad that I would sometimes take long naps in an effort to try to avoid the pain.

Shortly after daddy died, there were times when I felt that I was having pains in my chest (maybe due to stress or indigestion).   Although I was never diagnosed with a heart problem, I experienced the same symptoms of pain in my chest before my daughter was born.

Of all things, I thought, "Oh God please, not cancer."

As an adult, chocolates, soft drinks, tea and too many sweets had dominated my diet. This had been my temporary solution for not being able to communicate my fears, loneliness, and doubts and even for celebrating good things that had happened in my life.   It was as if I traded sweets for not drinking, not smoking, and for not using illegal drugs.

One weekend, while I was in college, I ate a pound of vanilla wafers and drank a quart of chocolate milk. I thought then I would die—I hurt so badly at 4:00 a.m. It was usually 4:00 a.m. that my sweet tooth had caused my stomach to ache, and I knew that it was always going to happen. My weakness for eating sweets had gotten me up at 4:00 a.m. almost crawling to the bathroom in pain more times than I can count.

My mother always had a problem with me taking medicine when I was little. It was nothing for me to drink a full eight-ounce glass of water to take one aspirin.   But—as an adult, Pepto-Bismol was a regular item in my grocery cart, and it usually worked wonders. Matter-of-fact, I only took Bayer Aspirin for headaches and Pepto-Bismol for stomach aches.

Regardless, ice tea and Coca Cola had almost taken the place of water in my daily liquid diet until I had to be treated for a kidney infection in 1974. I would drink six to eight small bottles of Coca Cola on Thursday nights (my usual all night cleaning night at home), not to mention the amount that I had already drank at work. Then when my son was born in 1977, for whatever reason, my taste for Coca Cola changed to the likes of Dr. Pepper.

In my work area, I usually sat next to co-workers who smoked. The Dallas County courthouse especially, where I worked for four years, was the home of cigar, pipe and cigarette haven. There was no way to escape the fumes.

My husband smoked in his truck but never in our house or in my car. So I rarely came in contact with his direct smoke except on his clothes or in his hair. Sometimes, at social gatherings though, the passive smoke in the room irritated my eyes.

I never smoked or drank, and since I had grown up in the country eating plenty of fresh garden vegetables and fruits, I hadn't worried about my health. Pinto beans and carrots had been my favorite vegetables. We had pork mostly when it came to meats, but there was always fresh milk, eggs and homegrown fruits and vegetables. My mother, to this day, says that I loved pinto beans so much that I could eat them for breakfast, dinner and supper.

Before daddy died of his heart attack, I remember long days in the cotton fields where the sun's rays felt like long hot switches burning through all the layers of clothing I wore. While chopping and picking cotton—talking about wishing for rain—a small cloud would seem like a miracle from heaven. After a while, my little brown gloves became worn, exposing my hands to wormy cotton stalks and blade-sharp grass, peeling the meat on the side of my little fingers. Sweat over my brow made my old hat itch my head and forehead. I couldn't stand being in the sun. It caused me to get so hot that my nose would bleed like tomato juice. I was eleven, but God was no stranger to me. We had a regular conversation.

Just the same, there I was sitting in awe as to why this had happened, and angry with myself that I had not come to the doctor sooner; angry that I had not taken better care of myself. A bill had always come first, or the children's needs, and since they were older—a sale item that I had been waiting for—and I just kept putting off my checkups.

Dr. Fosmire finished reviewing the lab work and his questions came next for me. How long had I felt the lump, was it sore, had there been any leakage from the breast, did I drink or smoke, and then the ultimate question—had I been examining myself? The word lump or mass had never entered my mind until he said it, and I still couldn't say it. I was referring to my breast as "the breast." I was trying to put some distance between the cancer and me any way that I could, and the only lump I could detect was the one in my throat right then.

I explained that the knot had been there for several months, only not as large and barely noticeable until I bumped it. Then I noticed the swelling and soreness.

Although there had not been any leakage from my breast, Dr. Fosmire inserted a needle to see if there was a fluid build-up. Instead, his first analysis after the chest x-ray and mammography was confirmed. Looking at the screen, the lump and the mass around it left little to be explained.

The next magical words that followed were heart breaking: lump, tumor, preliminary test, hospital, surgery, and mastectomy. Dr. Fosmire explained that I needed the surgery sooner than I expected.

"Lord, please, not yet," I thought.

I felt that there had to be another answer and what I needed most was something that I was running out of—time.

My heart just seemed to have stopped, and the only things still going on were the tears running down my face. The time felt right to throw in the towel, but I just couldn't say the words.

"Ok, so what, I have cancer. I've got to die sometimes." I just kept thinking. "Sometimes, but not right now Lord!"

I wanted to walk away and pretend that this day had never happened, but I had to remember because it was my tomorrow that I had prayed to see thirty years ago when my father died.

At my father's funeral, I remember reading on the program that he was forty-two. At twelve, I was awfully afraid of dying. I had prayed that I would at least live to be forty-two, and according to my prayers, my time was just about up. I wondered if God had answered yes or no. I wondered if God had answered at all. Even if it were just nine more days before my 42nd birthday, surely God hadn't brought me this close to say no; surely not.

I felt so nervous and upset by then that I just sat tearful, listening to Dr. Fosmire. When he finished talking to me about the exam, he told me to think about what I was going to do. In the meantime, Dr. Fosmire's secretary made the appointment for me to come in again on the following Monday.

I was frustrated, and no matter what had caused the cancer, everything around me seemed to say, "I did it!"

I was paranoid. For the past ten years, I had sat in front of a word processor or a computer screen, and now I wondered if the screen had given off too much radiation. The comfort, if there was any, was that I really enjoyed my work, and the key to going on was not to look back without remembering that. I had received two certificates in Word Processing, and I had truly enjoyed the climb up to my position as secretary in my division; not to mention that I had received a substitute teacher's certificate which I had planned to use once I retired from the City.

The next morning when I went to work, it must have registered on my face that all of this was still on my mind. I told my division manager, Barbara Reading, that my visit to the doctor was one of unexpectedly bad news. The subject was so overwhelming that I asked to be excused until later to explain.

Not knowing the situation, but seeing that I was obviously upset, Barbara was very understanding. She only replied, "Yes. Are you ok Earlene?"

I said yes and went to my desk. I had always had a smile on my face in the morning; not a lot to say, but at least a smile. Not this morning. Under the circumstances, it was difficult to focus on my job duties, and it became increasingly difficult as time progressed to keep my composure.

Jerry Darden, a Surveyor in the department, came by my desk—and as usual—he said good morning. I barely looked up or managed to say anything before I was in tears. He asked what was wrong, and I explained that I had gotten a bad report from my doctor.

Jerry said, "Come on and walk with me down the hall."

He asked me if I believed in God, and we talked about my church membership, trust and faith in God. Then he took my hand and prayed. Before walking me back to my desk, Jerry assured me that he would keep me in his prayers. He insisted, however, that I call my pastor, Reverend Smith at Ebenezer Baptist Church.

When I finally called Reverend Smith, he was out of town. I never called him back; neither did I leave a message for him to call me back. It was difficult to talk to anyone about what was happening to me. I just couldn't understand why God had allowed this to happen.

Jerry didn't know me very well then even though we worked in the same department, but I was grateful that he had taken the time to listen and pray with me.

The following Monday, February 11, I went back to see Dr. Fosmire. He scheduled the biopsy for that next week on Monday at 7:00 a.m.

With all of the pressures from just waiting, I knew that my strength had to have come from a supreme power. In spite of all of my fears, I felt that if God was going to leave me, he had passed over many opportunities to do so; when the children were small or when my marriage was in trouble. Even before all of that, when daddy died and two months later my baby brother—my playmate—died, when my nephew was brutally murdered, and while I was in the operating room all the times before, God's mercy still prevailed. These thoughts were comforting because in my present status, God had given me Jerry to stand where my little brother might have stood with me and the rest of my family. Jerry told me that God always sent a comforter, and he was sure right.

On Monday, February 18th, my sister Lois drove me to the Dallas Medical and Surgical Clinic for the biopsy. Dr. Fosmire had been delayed, but everything else was on schedule. I was taken to the operating room, the I.V. was started, and my arms were strapped in place for the surgery. The anesthesiologist talked to me about how I felt and then he explained what was going to take place. He talked to me about the medication to be administered, and he confirmed that I had followed his instructions—nothing to eat or drink since midnight before the scheduled operation.

As the medication started to take affect, I became drowsy and sleepy, but I could hear the medical staff wondering out-loud if Dr. Fosmire had been called away to the hospital for an emergency.

I thought, "I hope not because I want to get this over with."

The nurses and the anesthesiologist continued to talk to me and to make me comfortable as we waited for Dr. Fosmire. The I.V. made me feel cold, but thank God for the nurse who brought me a warm blanket.

"Thank you, thank you so much! That is much better. Thank you." I mumbled.

When Dr. Fosmire arrived, the anesthesiologist administered the appropriate amount of medication for my I.V. which must have taken affect immediately. The last thing I remember was one of the nurses saying, "Here's Dr. Fosmire," and Dr. Fosmire coming over to talk to me.

When the procedure was done, as expected, it was malignant. After a brief recovery period, with help from the nurse and Lois, I was able to dress myself and get into a wheelchair for the distance to my sister's car. I was still sedated, but I could feel the tenderness from the incision where the stitches were.

I didn't have any questions for Dr. Fosmire. He had always explained very thoroughly the next step. He emphasized that time was of utmost importance—that nothing had changed.

I knew that I had a long and difficult week ahead of me. It would be difficult because I was still in denial of how necessary the operation was, and I was still hoping that further testing would overrule the results of previous tests. In reality, it was already definite that the operation was a must. Words like lump, tumor, operation and mastectomy had come up at every doctor's visit. Knot was clearly a forgotten word.

I wished this had been the major surgery, and with that on my mind, I didn't talk very much on the way home.

I went in the next day to see Dr. Fosmire for my follow-up and continued instructions for further scheduled test. Dr. Fosmire didn't waste time. He scheduled the bone and liver test for the following morning at 9:30 a.m. in the Jonsson Hospital Unit at Baylor Hospital. He also asked me if I wanted to get a second opinion. When I said yes, he recommended Dr. Knox, a female doctor.

"Oh thank God," I thought. "She will tell him that there is another alternative "

And—for that moment, I was feeling better. Dr. Fosmire emphasized how important it was for me to get in to see Dr Knox as soon as possible. Before I headed for home, Linda, Dr. Fosmire's nurse—called to set up the appointment for me.

The next morning, February 20th, Lois took me over to Baylor for the bone and liver test. After I had registered and sat down, I noticed a sign that read "Pay as you are being served." I didn't have enough money to pay for the service.

"How, or what am I going to do?" I thought.

This added to my stress. Finally I walked to the service desk and told the administrator that I couldn't pay for the services. She looked up and smiled.

"Don't worry about that, we'll see if your insurance covers it. You just come on in when you're called. We'll take care of that later."

I was glad to get the test behind me, thinking that it was just another confirmation that I had cancer. Instead, when the testing was completed, it was confirmation that the cancer had not spreaded to my liver and bones. God really was working it out.

Lois drove me home, and as usual, she asked, "Do you need me to do anything else?"

Short of a healing miracle, I couldn't think of anything.

The next day, February 21, 1991, I went alone to see Dr. Knox in the Burnette Tower building at Baylor Hospital for my second opinion consultation. She examined me and discussed the report with me. It was basically the same as Dr. Fosmire's report. However, I was more prepared this time to hear the words lump, tumor and mass, but I still wanted to hear an alternative to the word mastectomy.

Dr. Knox explained that the lump and the mass surrounding it had grown too large to even tamper with the risk of not having the mastectomy. When she had explained everything and answered what few questions I had left, Dr. Knox asked if she could pray with me. I was still very nervous and weak, but the prayer was comforting. Plus, it was good hearing these things from a woman.

On my way home, I tried to accept fully that the two doctors were right; that they really were trying to help me. Yet all of this was a lot to grasp in such a short time, and it certainly took a lot of energy just trying to get through even an hour at a time.

When I went back to work, my division manager, Barbara Reading and one of the other engineers, Alberta Blair-Robinson, sat with me and walked with me to help me get through the long days before surgery. And—Jerry Darden kept his promise. He kept calling and he kept praying with me.

Then I guess pretty soon, everyone in my division was encouraging me to keep my chin up.

When I went home, I cried for my family— especially for my children. Lester Jr. had been diagnoses with asthma when he was two years old. We had taken him to the hospital in the middle of the night so many times before when his little inhaler that his doctor prescribed wasn't enough to get his breathing under control. Most nights he could not sleep, and when he went to school he usually slept through his classes. Before we knew it, he was missing his basic studies and having problems keeping up in his classes. He continued to sleep in kindergarten and throughout most of his early grades until he was placed in Special Education. Marfa and Lester Jr. were opposites. She had gotten her basics and learned well, but he had not. By age thirteen, Lester Jr. seemed more embarrassed, and he didn't want anyone to know what he didn't know. Children were poking fun and always bringing it to his attention that he was still having problems with basic things like simple math, reading, writing, telling time and counting money. Who would be there for my children to lean on? These were new beginnings for both of them. My son was just turning thirteen and my daughter had just graduated from high school. What a decision for a high school graduate? Was she to continue her education or go to work fulltime? In addition—Lester Jr. needed me too. I begged God for mercy—for life. I wanted God's promise that he would be everything they needed in my absence.

Lester Sr. had not been able to fully accept the challenges we faced with our son. He seemed to have had no idea what to do for Lester Jr. sometimes, but he held on to his hopes that Lester Jr. would overcome some limits regardless of what his teachers said. He simply gave him anything that he thought he needed or wanted for that matter; his reason being that he had not had many of the things that he needed or wanted as a child himself, but Lester Sr. had learned his basics. Lester Sr. could read and write and make reasonable decisions by himself. In the meantime, Lester Jr. wanted to make his father proud of him, and he often tried to mimic him. Lester Sr. even tried to teach Lester Jr. some of the things that he had missed in school. Since Lester Jr. could walk, he and his father had been inseparable. Lester Sr. often took Lester Jr. along when he went to do plumbing repair jobs which he learned very well.

I cried too, because of more personal reasons. I didn't want the operation to take place because of so many other fears. I had so many questions. What did my family expect from me? Why couldn't I just give God back my life and forget about surgery? I wondered if I could accept the difference in my life and go on in positive ways. My biggest fear was that others would overlook my inside and whisper more about my outside. I cried for moments that I felt I would never know again—to be held and loved by a special man in my life who would understand and have the same love for me that I would for him.

I cancelled such words as men, love and marriage, and in exchange, I adopted such words as doubts, fears and loneliness. Only, it was still decision time, and I couldn't just give up since God had the last word. I had to trust him.

Looking back, on two marriages that ended in divorce, I had learned that being married was not a cure for loneliness or any of the other things that I was feeling. Even the children were not always a cure for those times, and they had been my company—my real pride and joy.

As time passed, the nights seemed longer, and I couldn't sleep, so I had to pray. Even though my bedroom door was closed, my son could hear me crying, and he would ask me if he could do anything. My heart went out to him for trying so hard to help, but I worried about what else he was thinking or if he was scared. I tried to explain to him that my being sick was not his fault, that I loved him, and that it was a lot of help just having him around.

While Lester Jr. spent more and more time with his father, my daughter seemed very distant. I gathered that it was a very frightening time for her, especially since she smoked. She tried to learn to do more and to be on her own. She even worked longer hours, and she spent more time to herself when she wasn't working. She didn't let me see her cry—if she did. One part of me understood her, but another part of me didn't. I wanted Marfa and Lester Jr. to be around more to help each other cope. Instead, it was the opposite, Marfa just went her separate way, and it seemed that we disagreed about everything. The isolation from her was very painful. I worried about her being on her owns, yet I needed to know that she could be without me. And—I imagined that she was trying to do just that.

Meanwhile, in my mind, I wondered if the doctors would catch the cancer in time. I wondered even more about what God's plans were for me. My prayers had grown from a word to a sentence and pretty soon, to a paragraph.

"Oh Dear God, should I get my coat now that you've checked me out? When I served you Lord, didn't you know that—that was my best? Is it just time Lord? Haven't I been a good parent? Sometimes I worked two jobs rather than turning to the wrong sources of support for my children. I helped my family. I helped some people that I didn't even know Lord—with compassion and love. If it's really time, I mean really time Lord—please take care of my children. Lord—I really do thank you for my life."

I prayed daily, not realizing that God's plan for me was beyond age 42; not realizing that God had graciously answered me with his blessings. I was not focusing on the fact that he had forbidden the cancer to go beyond the mass. I was not focusing on the fact that he had hidden my bones from the diseased messenger or that he had protected the rest of me from death's trapped doors. So I begged God's mercy, and I waited with a dimmer faith at my side.

Chapter 2

Is the Mission Impossible?

On Tuesday, February 26, 1991, ten days after my 42nd birthday at 8:00 a.m., I was admitted to the Hobilitzelle Unit of Baylor Hospital, in Dallas Texas. Dr. George P. Fosmire and his medical team performed the modified radical mastectomy.

For me, it was a personal and private walk down the hall to my room. Trading stories like mine or worst didn't seem to fit my schedule that day. I felt weak—reason enough to pray: "Precious Lord, would you please take my hand?"

I was tired and weak from waiting, and it was time to get on with the operation. I had been awake most of the night before, just thinking and praying.

Meanwhile, the room was clean and as accommodating as any hospital room could be. From the window, to my right, I could see a small portion of downtown Dallas. To my left, from the same window, memories of happier days filled my mind as I stood reminiscing and admiring the beautiful sky over the South Dallas Fair Park area. I don't know what the weather was like that day. I just know that to me, it was a beautiful day. A bit closer, outside the window on the roof, was the landing space for the hospital's emergency helicopter.

Life just seemed to have stared me in my face, and the opportunities that stood with it offered me a much closer look at myself. Yet, I questioned this wonderful dream of time—something that I had often taken for granted. It was obviously a moment to identify my own peacemaker; a time to shout from the inside:

"Father, I stretch my hands to thee. There's no other help I know."

It was the perfect time to thank God for sustaining me through all of my weakness, and for turning all of my midnights into days. It was time to surrender all and to be grateful that there was hope. It was time to forgive myself, and time to listen to life's conductor:'

"Going my way?"

As I recall, shortly after settling in my room, I was given a hospital gown and cap, vitals were checked and the I.V. was started. The medication took affect immediately, and I vaguely remember being taken to the operating room.

My memory does not serve me adequately in remembering how long it took or how long I was in recovery, but I am told that the surgery took several hours and that I was in recovery for sometime after that.

When I woke up, I was back in my room where I must have slept most of the afternoon until some of the staff came to check on my progress. Even then, I was only awake long enough to eat the soup brought in on my tray—with my sister's help—God permitting.

I was still heavily sedated, so I didn't remember much of anything about that afternoon. I was sleepy and tired, but I knew that the operation was over. For the rest of the evening and throughout the night, I slept comfortably. I was not alert enough to concern myself with how I looked. I was just glad that the operation was over and that God had answered my prayers and sustained my life.

I was more alert the next morning although, somewhat less sedated, and I wasn't sure where I was hurting most. The I.V. was still in my left wrist, and since I am right handed, it felt awkward to move. However, the drainage tube inserted during the surgery—and ironically—a part of me that wasn't there anymore all seemed to have been hurting.

Like the I.V., the tube was taped in place and there was minimum movement if any. A small sterile suction bulb was attached to the tube to collect excess fluid accumulated under my skin. The bulb was pinned to a wide white dressing that graced the upper swollen portion of my chest.

I was afraid to even entertain the idea of turning over. Whenever I tried to move, I felt instant distribution of torturous pain and an awfully stubborn numbness under my right arm. I was cold and nervous too—causing unintentional movement and consequently causing more pain. However, the soft white pillows that surrounded my right side and the warm blankets on the hospital bed were a welcomed attempt to pacify my tender discomforts. My bed was elevated to an upward position while I was being examined and refreshed. It seemed like a miracle just to be able to move enough to slowly eat some of my breakfast with help.

Again that afternoon, I was awake long enough to eat with help, and I was able to talk briefly to those who visited

19

me: my sister and co-workers Barbara Reading, Alberta Robinson, Tom Berry, Jerry and Thelma Darden. When they left, the TV in my room kept me company as I drifted off to sleep following my evening dose of pain medication.

I woke up the next morning to a new set of pains.

"I should feel better," I thought.

Only there were mental as well as physical pains. My past, present and future seemed to have been colliding—causing a very self-centered and confusing state of mind. Again, I blamed everything that might have remotely been capable of causing the cancer. I felt misplaced and detached from everything around me.

The hospital staff was at my bedside asking me questions.

"How do you feel? Are you in much pain? Can you try to sit up? Would you like some breakfast?"

And—it didn't matter what the answers were, because whenever I tried to move, everything seemed to have been hurting inside and out. The medication was making me drowsy and sleepy too. My balance was off, and I felt terribly weak. The taste of medication seemed to have sank deeper in my mind than in my mouth. I had no desire or taste for food although I was hungry. I just wanted an instant repair kit that would give me back my simple feeling for life.

The nurse left my tray with me in hopes that I would eat, but when my daughter came to see me, I offered her portions of my food. It seemed such a waste that I wasn't going to eat all of it.

I prayed that Dr. Fosmire was right, even though he had been right two times before. Only this was the most pain that I had ever known—even compared to childbirth. I just wanted to

20

lie there in that hospital bed and not have to get up—and surely not have to witness anymore physical or emotional pain. I didn't want anyone to see me until I could get my emotions in order.

I begged God's mercy for my attitude, but I prayed more for the patience of the hospital staff—that they would not give up on me. I prayed that they could understand how much pain I was in.

I couldn't lift my hand to touch my face without being in severe pain. Lymph nodes had been removed from under my right arm, and it felt very stiff and numb to touch. Comparatively, missing a nail and hitting one's finger while hammering may best attempt to describe the lingering pain.

The pain in my upper body seemed unbearable. Around the surgical area, stitches were in a half circle starting from the middle of my chest ending just inside my armpit. My armpit felt as if it was being stretched and reversed—ripping the stitches out—opening up the surgical area.

I pleaded with God, "Oh Lord, please, have mercy. Please Jesus!"

The staff was prepared more than I for my physical limitations, but it was evident that I was more afraid of what was yet to come. They sensed my emotional pain, and assured me that everything was progressing as well as expected. Nonetheless, in my mind, Dr. Fosmire was the best surgeon on earth, but if he couldn't fix me up right, God just must not have intended for me to be fixed up.

Regardless of how optimistic I tried to be, after seeing the two holes that had been drilled into my side, where the drainage tube was inserted, I started to experience even more stress. There were so many contradictions in my mind. I had endless questions as to why I couldn't move my right arm past my ear without extreme pain.

"How long Lord, will I be in this much pain? Will I ever be able to fully use my arm again? Only you can help Lord!" This was my daily prayer.

Although, Dr. Fosmire emphasized that the surgery had gone well, my expectations just didn't match his. I had no earthly idea how I was going to get myself out of bed or even remotely how I was going to raise up. The pain was a constant reminder—like bolts of lighting finding all of my bones in their hiding places—beneath my chilled skin, touching and draining my strength. Inborn fears came from storage places somewhere in my brain and surfaced so often that I could think of nothing but the intense pain of that moment.

If I used my arm on the operative side for support, my chest would hurt as if the two-day-old stitches were being branded into my chest right then. It was like waking up in the middle of the operation feeling tender cuts; a nightmare where thick broken glass or a razor blade was being used to tear out my breast from under my skin, and than an anchor or weight put in its place.

Meanwhile, trying to use my left hand, where the I.V. was inserted, alerted me to the frightening thoughts of slipping and falling down, causing the I.V. to sink deeper into my raw skin. Such intense pain placed me in a semiconscious state of mind, yet it was more than a simple reminder that the gift of life was still spreading itself plentifully throughout my body.

I had to talk to God. In light of the pain, I had to begin a positive thought process. I had to overcome my panic-stricken ideas—that the numbness and the pain were all over my body. My arm was more sore than I expected. Prior to the surgery when Dr. Fosmire had explained the procedure, I had only remembered four words: lump, cancer, surgery and mastectomy. The rest of that conversation had lingered cold in my mind.

Consequently, I was continuing to experience such mental and emotional stress that it seemed to out-weigh the physical pain. Not only that, I was beginning to think that I had asked God for the wrong thing—to spare my life. I was having a hard time believing and trusting God's power. The pain was so distracting that I focused on my own sufferings and timid thoughts.

"Don't you see me Lord? Don't you know how much pain I'm in? Is this mission impossible?"

I felt like the disciples on board the ship with Jesus when the storm started to rage, as Jesus slept. I wanted to ask him just as they did, "Master carest thou not?"

I tried to remember what Dessie Minor had said before the operation: "God is not the author of confusion, and God surely keeps his promises."

But Lord, I sure felt plenty of confusion—so much that—I was pleading, "Lord please be faithful in your word. You know how much I can really stand. Lord, if you're really up there, and you are listening to my fainting plea—Oh Dear God, please—please, please help me Lord.

I was in so much pain that nothing else was left but to call on God. The doctors had done their part, the nurses were still helping me, but in a few days, I would be going home to double duty to help myself.

My mind pondered questions that I knew only God could answer. "What if I fell and couldn't get up? What if I couldn't move my arm well enough to empty the fluid? What if I became infected? How could I keep from getting a cold; especially a coughing cold or worst—pneumonia? What would I have to take to get better? Would I have to go back to the hospital? Would I see my children grow up? Would I just get infected this time and die?

Dessie had said that we all need to stay prayed up. Finally I knew exactly what she meant. How soon—if at all-would a better tomorrow come along?

I prayed, "Wake me up one morning soon Lord—with amazement in my heart—knowing that I have survived; that your grace and mercy really did prevail."

I cried for unknown fears, I prayed for strength, and finally I cried for God's goodness. I started to remember the prior surgery when the fibroid tumors were removed. I had gone home from the hospital with staple stitches then, and I remember thinking that I had felt nothing as sensitive as that pain. I could not bend or walk up straight the first few days home from the hospital. I was in so much pain then that I didn't take the chance on not believing in God. Again, in my heart, I was reminded that this was no time to become a-none believer.

I was remembering past and present pain so much, that I was afraid to get of the hospital bed. However, I was about to learn a lot of things, including more patience with myself and a lot more faith in God.

The nurse asked me if I felt up to going to therapy, and in my mind, the answer was overwhelmingly no—with tears that rendered me speechless at first.

I didn't respond with my thoughts though: "Now just how am I expected to go to therapy if I can't even hold my little plastic eating utensil or a small plastic container of juice? I can't even open a small paper milk carton to insert a straw. I don't possess an ounce of strength to unpin the little bulb attached to my beloved little dressing without being in tremendous silly pain. How am I expected to get up Lord? When I try to reach, my body is too weak and the pain is too much. It seems that the pillows slip away like melted butter sticks when I try to raise myself up using them for support!"

So, I continued to ask God, "Don't you see me Lord?" Please—please have mercy. I don't think that I can do this."

Well, despite all of my pitiful little thinking and mental anguish, and much to my surprise, my thoughts were surely going to change. This, at first, felt like a major humiliation. Did they really think that I could sit in a counseling session without crying my eyes out, without excruciating pain, and without becoming more tired?

Furthermore, I didn't want anyone to see me. I was thinking more about how I looked, and my self-esteem was immeasurably low. I didn't know what to expect, and my reply was, "Do I really have to do this today?"

I was hoping that the nurse would say that if I didn't feel up to it, I could wait until the next day. Instead, she answered, "Yes you do. You really will feel better."

Without voicing further complaints, I agreed to go to therapy, and I prayed that I could just do what I was being asked to do. The staff was so persistent that I started to wonder if I really was ok.

I was so nervous and cold that I couldn't distinguish the pain from the fear. I dreaded going to a counseling session where everyone was in terrible pain, frightening me more with their stories, being told that life was going to be such a beautiful little bed of roses, and that ahead of me would be such a big romantic challenge.   Nor did I feel up to viewing films, listening to tapes or playing what if games.   This was very private to me.   I didn't want to discuss it with people that I didn't know or with people who had never even had cancer or an I.V. in their healthy little risk.

I felt so upset with God.   I was beginning to wonder how I could lean on someone that I couldn't even trust.   I felt so confused.   I was angry because I needed help, but I was weak and unable to do almost everything without help.   I still couldn't lift my hand up to my face to even wipe the tears without severe pain.

Just the same, I listened to the nurse for further instructions.   Then she gently helped me out of bed, and slowly I was on my feet.   The pain was awesome, I was weak, and I felt dizzy, but I was so happy that I could stand.   The nurse was right.   Before, I had become so panic-stricken that I was ready to give up.

I will forever thank God for the staff at Baylor—for their professional gifts in the medical field—especially for their patience and persistence.   When the nurse helped me down the hall, I really felt that God had granted me some reassurance that I was going to be all right.

The therapy session consisted of a volunteer and a member of the hospital staff.   Their smiles, as they greeted me and reached for my hand, again assured me of God's everlasting mercy.   There were no films, no tapes, and no crowds.   It was a very private and personal session.

The volunteer said, "I know what you're going through."

She continued to talk to me, and I learned that she had experienced far more pain than I had.   She talked with such kindness and comforting words.   She expressed so much enthusiasm for life, and she listened to what little I had to say. She and the counselor answered questions that I didn't even know how to ask. They understood my tears, my fears, my anger, my frustrations, my sorrows, and pity for myself, but most of all—my strong will to live.

I listened with tears, for the strength and joy they shared—that God could be so good; that God had allowed me this chance to know that I wasn't along in my sufferings.

Weeping had endured through so many nights before and after the surgery, and someone very strong was bearing the infirmities of my weakness. Jerry and Dessie were right again. God had always sent a comforter. He always had someone for me when I really needed them most.

The volunteer counselor told me how she had survived a double mastectomy, and now how she was enjoying her life to the fullest. Her husband and her family had given her special love and moral support.

She really could say, "I know how you feel."

I couldn't equate the same, on a personal level, about my husband since we were divorced. I don't remember him even bringing our children to see me while I was in the hospital after this surgery, and I couldn't imagine ever going through all of this again. Yet there I was listening to the counselors telling me not to shut out others close to me; how to accept love and support from others who were there for me. They were explaining how to let God work through their staff, as well as through my own family and some special friends, who would help me get through my fears.

I felt God's word fulfilled in his promise. He had made it possible for me to still receive my blessings in the middle of what felt to be the biggest storm of my life.

Dessie had repeatedly told me, "Whatever God has for you, you're going to get it sugar, but you can't hurry him."

I don't remember just how long the session lasted—thirty-five, forty minutes or maybe an hour—but when it was over, my thoughts were more positive. I also had some idea of what to expect. I only hoped that my family would be patient and understanding. I prayed that I could be more patient with myself and that I could be thankful for any progress that I made.

I could barely move or sit without pain, and I was tired. So I was glad to get back to my room. I started to accept the result of the operation that would change some parts of my life forever. I tried to leave some thoughts behind as well so that I could get on with helping myself. I started to think more instead of complaining. I realized too, that I had more hills to climb than I had already surpassed. My own fears had been enough to keep me at the bottom. So little by little, some of my fears were also left behind, and I found myself more receptive and grateful that so many people were around.

In the meantime, I had some time to rest before lunch. So I put everything aside and just watched TV. I rehearsed in my mind how I was going to dress myself. I got up to go to the bathroom on my own, and slowly I was able to adjust my bed pillows. I even talked to my family and co-workers on the phone.

Later that afternoon, more of my family visited: my aunt Betty, uncle Prentis, and my niece Vickie. My brother Eddie and his wife Elouise had sent me a cute little plant, and my oldest sister Clarine sent me a card that further touched my heart and gave me encouragement. I read that card over and over again. Up to that point, everyone in my family had come or responded except my mother. My sister was going to pick her up later since it was nearing my release to go home, but she hadn't said anything and I was starting to wonder why. My mother would have been the first to call and come if she had to pay someone to bring her. Finally they told me that mother was also in the hospital for chest pains in Greenville, Texas. Although mother was resting comfortably by the time they told me, I worried that they had not told me the whole story since she was in intensive care. Little was said to me, only that she might have suffered a heart attack.   I was grateful for medication that made me sleep so that I wouldn't be awake to think.

I had another visitor that evening, my sister-in-law, Ruby. As usual, she checked on my children. She seemed more like a sister than a sister-in-law. She tried to help Lester Sr. all she could with Lester Jr. and Marfa.

When my sister-in-law left, that same afternoon, I had another unexpected visitor. It was Debbie McDonald, the Cancer Society's volunteer from their Reach to Recovery Program. She had a little bag for me which included a small pillow that she had tucked into a little blue pillowcase, a temporary breast form, and some helpful reading material that described the program and its purpose.   The information contained in the reading material provided information on breast reconstruction, types of permanent prostheses and a list of retailers who could fit me with the prostheses as well as an adjustable bra, if I chose not to have the breast reconstruction surgery. One of the shops recommended was a little shop right there at the hospital in the Komen building. The booklet also gave specific exercises and other helpful hints and 'how to' for helpful grooming ideas; scarves, hats, bras, and clothing styles etc. Counseling programs were a part of the information for patients once discharged from the hospital also. Debbie talked with me for a few minutes, but before she left, she gave me her calling card which read: "For what you have done in other days and for what you will do today, I give thanks, Oh Lord. Amen."

I counted heavily on the later part of that little message.

Later, Dessie Minor—one of our mission teachers from my church also came by that day. She had such a positive spirit. "How you doing sugar? God is able," she said.

Dessie stayed just a little while, and before she left, she prayed with me. Her hand was in a cast, but she didn't once complain about pain, driving or any other obstacle that might have caused a problem for her coming to the hospital that day. I was just glad that she remembered that I was there and that she took the time to come by to see me.

One more visitor would come before Dr. Jones, the Oncologist. Orr Hinton, another co-worker who was an Inspector in the Public Works Department where I worked came by. He was there only a few minutes before Dr. Jones came in to talk to me. Dr. Jones asked Orr if he would wait outside my room while he visited with me.

It was during that visit with Dr. Jones that I was made aware that I would needed chemotherapy treatments. I had been so busy worrying about my "right now situation," and I was focusing so much on what had already happened, that I hadn't thought about the follow-up treatments. Further-to-that, even after Dr. Jones had explained about the treatments, I didn't completely understand, and I was wondering if I would need radiation too.

30

After his visit, Dr. Jones invited Orr back to complete his visit with me. I was upset by this news and experiencing a lot of 'Why God' feelings, but I was reminded of something that Dessie Minor had said, "God always sends somebody."

Had I been alone in that hospital room when Dr. Jones left, I would have just sat and cried. I was still in a lot of pain, and this news didn't help.

I don't recall what I said when Orr came back into the room, but I was so grateful that he stayed. He was company when I really needed a smile from a friend. He made me laugh and forget long enough to get control of my fears. I sat there trying not to seem upset, grateful that I wasn't alone to think about the treatment.

When Orr left, watching his car pull away from the parking lot, I thanked God for his visit. Someone had always been around at the most sensitive times. Dessie and Jerry always reminded me that God knew how much I could bear.

When the day ended, I slept through the night, and after several days, it was finally time to go home.

Again, my sister Lois was there to help me check out and to take me home. The worst seemed to be over, and I welcomed the seat in a wheelchair—a very careful ride from the lady in white. My sister walked beside us carrying some of my things, as the nurse pushed me out to her car. I looked back only to say good-by to overwhelming memories of tears and limited laughter. Yet, on the contrary, my look back greeted blessed moments that only God could have handled through the Baylor staff of caretakers, and I was able to smile in the middle of all my pain. I was able to smile with all of the staff members who smiled and wished me well. The medication had not voided all of my pain, but I knew from their smiles that bigger blessings were somewhere ahead.

Recovery was about to introduce itself, and again I was reminded of my own peacemaker—my real company keeper. It was a moment inside that addressed my feelings clearly. I was remembering the words of a hymn: "I love the Lord. He heard my cry and pitted my every groan." As we drove off, I didn't think much more about anything. I wanted to just keep on praying because that was the only way I felt that I would be all right. I didn't want to cry in front of Lois anyway. She drove as careful as she could. Now, I sometimes smile and even laugh aloud at how careful she tried to be that day. She had been such a blessing to have around.

Chapter 3

Order My Steps Lord

It was close to noon or shortly thereafter when my sister and I arrived at my house. She got my prescriptions and helped me settle in before she left.

I was glad that my children weren't home yet. Although it was difficult to help myself, I felt that I needed that time alone to pray. I needed some time to pray that I could accept my weaknesses and realize my potential strengths. This had been a long week for me, and as strange as it all seemed, it really was good to be home.

Reviewing life's cards as they had been dealt to me, I toured the house like it was my first time. Remembering, if I had not rounded that corner from the living room and banged myself on the kitchen wall, I might not have been alive to notice such vivid details around me. Better yet, I might not have been around to even focus on the little things to come in my life.

Gently, I reach out to touch the wall that—through God's love and mercy—had ironically given me life. The textured surface revealed a thin bladed paralytic edge, equal in my mind, to the strength of steel. It was sophisticatedly hidden underneath the off-white paint. The craftsmanship, of a coarse but gracefully wrinkled effect, reminded me of my rough path to recovery.

From my patio door, I witnessed little birds sitting on the edge of the wood fence, and around the yard—nature's symbols of spring all dressed up in its green attire. I felt so much loose pride just waiting to be nurtured back into its respective place. Right then, I wanted to be like the birds that sat confidently on the edge of the wood fence—without hesitation. I wanted that confidence, and I wanted desperately to find my way back to just being my old self again.

Only, there was no old. Everything looked and felt completely new, and at times—strangely uncomfortable. The house was clean and refreshing. Yet the absence of the hospital staff reminded me that there was no panic button to push; that I was very much on my own.

I knew that my children wouldn't know what to expect. They wouldn't understand my limitations. My daughter may have had a better idea than my son about what had already happened, but neither one had a clue as to what to expect from me emotionally.

In the meantime, reality was starting to feel like a head-on collision. Moving around was breathtakingly slow--tediously slower than I expected. The little things that had always come so natural and easy were major task. Little children didn't have to climb up or reach for items—that seemed—unreachable for me.

Praying that I would not slip and fall, I held on to whatever was closest to me as I walked. The drainage tube in my right side was uncomfortable enough that I always remembered that it was there. The sore upper part of me made lifting my hand to my face a five-minute task. I knew that if the phone rang, it would take real gutbucket nerve to get up or attempt to reach for it.

It was a moaning and tearful experience facing the reality that I had such a long way to go; that a number of other things were on hold as well. Housework in general was one of them, including the simple chore of dusting. To swing my arm back and forth, up and down, and surely in any circular motion was not going to happen as soon as I had hoped without extreme pain.

When I got to the kitchen sink, I found that I didn't have the strength to turn on the faucet. Furthermore, it was extremely painful trying to bend or reach up into the kitchen cabinet, pick up dishes, open the refrigerator or to even open a small cereal box. And—if by chance—I wasted something, I couldn't clean it up.

As I glanced down the hall into my bedroom, I knew too, that making my bed, hanging my clothes—all called for help. I didn't want any help doing these things. I just wanted God to give me back my strength; my tomorrow. It wasn't easy to pray without questions, but it was easy to pray.

It was starting to be a very frightening experience. I think I realized then what the elderly and handicapped persons must go through on a daily basis. More so, since I wore glasses, I could imagine the frustration of blind people (trying from day to day) and being ignored or mistreated (whether intentional or not) by those of us who can see. It was more of an obstacle to put my glasses on my face than trying to make out the scenes around me due to my blurred vision.

As I continued to walk through the house and into the bathroom—a routine last stop—the mirror reminded me of a stranger. Staring into that mirror and seeing the surgical area, I felt so much stress and emotional pain; equal, if not worst, to the physical pain. I pulled the lid down on the toilet seat, sat slowly and just cried:

"Oh Dear God! Oh my Dear God! Oh God please!"

I don't know how long I sat, but I probably cried harder than I had ever cried before. Right then my only question to God was, "Oh God, why has this happened to me?"

I was overwhelmed with grief, and there was no acceptance. My faith was totally consumed by my grief. I was thinking more about how I looked. Not only that, I was terrified by the thought of the chemotherapy treatments.

I had cried so hard that my mouth was extremely dry, and my back as well as the operative area was hurting worst. The kitchen seemed a mile away. Finally, after realizing that somehow, I had to get myself a drink of water, I stopped crying and started trying to figure out how I was going to function.

"Ok, I'm not blind. I'm not totally disabled. So I'll just have to get up faster." I thought.

Only, it wasn't that simple. When I started to get up, I met the resistance of razor sharp pains.

I pleaded with God continuously, "Please don't let me be so afraid that I can't help myself."

Taking my medicine, attending the healing area and accepting the reality—even for a start—seemed to be such a long list.

Although my sister would be back, I had to help myself right then. I managed to get back to my bedroom and to pour myself a glass of water from the little plastic water pitcher that I had brought home from the hospital. I tried to think positive.

"Earlene, this is not the time to give up; loose hope for trial and error and then no recovery." I thought.

Yet, I couldn't imagine how to begin recovery. All I wanted to do was sleep. I slept for about two hours, and I woke up to pain that kept me awake for two more hours; the beginning of unusual sleeping patterns. In addition to the pain, my upper body felt tightly swollen and sore, and my right under arm still felt numb. To further complicate things, my body was tired and aching from having lain in the same position too long. To get up I had to turn from my left side, using my left hand to lift my legs out of bed one at a time. I balanced myself while gripping my bedpost. All of this reminded me of the sensations that I initially felt after the operation, and it made me wish for the hospital staff to take care of me.

I don't remember much more about that day or night. I don't even remember what time my sister and my children came back. The medication was strong enough to relieve the pain, and I just slept.

The fear of torn stitches, congestion in my chest or a coughing cold causing painful movement and more aches and pain, infection or pneumonia, and bleeding—to mention a few—registered in my mind as often as my eyes opened. I woke up crying because I didn't know where I was hurting or if the pain was normal. Each time I prayed that the pain would just go away.

After several nights at home, I was getting around better, but my sleeping patterns were a bowl of confusion. However, I was learning to adjust. Being able to get to the bathroom and to do minor things for myself was a goal that I had to master. I didn't wake my children because I had to get better by doing for myself. My sick time and vacation time was running out at work. I had to learn how to accept my situation and get back to basics. Marfa was working, but she couldn't pay all the bills.

I had to keep telling myself that God wouldn't put more on me than I could stand, especially when the children weren't around. I had to learn how to accept help from others around me. And—God must have opened so many doors. The love and special time devoted to helping me recover by so many special people will forever be a memorial in my heart.

My first week home, I received numerous calls and visits from my family and co-workers, some of which I was quiet surprised to get.

Wanda Joe and Linda Gleghorn, from Public Works Administration, came by to visit me and to complete paperwork for on-going benefits. They asked what I needed—specifically what I needed to eat. I explained that I needed green vegetables, among other things. Well, I didn't take it to mean much beyond getting the paperwork done and a step up from curiosity or pity when they asked, especially since I didn't really know them. Besides, I wasn't in their division.

Nevertheless, God must have been listening to my heart and not the doubts in my mind. I had mounting utility bills and rent that I had no idea how I was going to continue to pay, and positive thinking wasn't at my fingertips.

A few days later, as a result of their visit and concerns, something very positive did happen. They sent Tom Berry, one of the inspectors from my division, out to bring me some green vegetables. I don't remember exactly what else was in the sacks, but I do remember that they had specifically shopped for foods that I had told them that I needed--and more importantly—foods that I could really prepare myself as the healing began. Tom also handed me an envelope that contained a get-well card, which included personal checks made out to me. It also included cash that totaled more than three hundred dollars. All of this had come from co-workers in all divisions of Public Works. Tom stood there a few minutes, giving me time to gather my composure. With his light touch, I don't think he knew whether to hug me or to just take my hand. Then he told me if I needed anything else to give some of them a call. I couldn't ask for more. Their time and love had given me hope that I could never have obtained by myself.

The following weekend, Modesta Pena, who was the secretary to the Director of Public Works, came by. She brought paper towel and a number of things—with her sleeves rolled up—ready to help me with housework. I couldn't believe that she had really come to do that. I really didn't know her either. A Saturday! She could have spent her time doing so many other things. Instead, when she came in, she just asked, "What can I do to help?"

As the weeks passed, just about everyone in my division had sent me a card or plant, came by to visit or called: Jerry Darden and his wife Thelma, Tom Berry, Orr Hinton, Barbara

Reading, Alberta Robinson with her mother and grandmother, Ron Crippens and his wife, Mike Heimlich and his wife, Bagwan Shah and his wife, Larry Smith and his wife, Ron Underwood and his wife, David White, Amrit Nigra, and Charolyn Sifford and her husband.

Charolyn Sifford and I had become lunch buddies after supervision for the Resurfacing Division of Public Works (where she worked) merged with the Central Business Division of Public Works (where I worked). She called daily and mailed me a number of cards with notes of encouragement for a healthy recovery. I still have her notes, and I sometimes laugh aloud when I read the messages on them.

Charolyn, Jerry and Orr called as much as my own family. There were some days when nothing seemed right, but they all helped me through the toughest hours.

My Aunt Betty came and brought me a month and more supply of grocery for the children and myself. She didn't cook, but we do share that phenomenon. We aren't the cooks in the family. I've often joked about that. Not that we can't! She worked long hours for AT&T, but she was in and out—always calling.

Some days, my sister-in-law Ruby cooked at her house, and brought food over. She seemed more like a sister than a sister-in-law. She was always coming by or calling to see what she could do to help.

Finally after a week and many calls, my mother did get to visit me. She had only been home from the hospital a few days herself, but she wasn't content until Lois brought her to see me. She was always asking if I was in pain, and my thinking cap was on automatic "no." I didn't want her to worry. I couldn't sit up a long time without pain, so I always told her that I was

40

just getting tired. By the time I got to my bedroom door, I was hurting so bad that I was in tears. I tried not to cry so that my eyes wouldn't be red because she noticed everything.

As the week progressed, I did get better, but not before experiencing more obstacles. To take a bath was probably the most difficult thing I had to do.   I was told to keep the operative area dry, and that meant covering the area with a plastic shield. I couldn't reach with the bath brush to wash my back, and I constantly dropped the soap. My mother was still visiting me, and I could hear her asking if I was all right. I was in pain, and it was hard to answer her in a clear voice.   I pretended not to hear her. Most of the time, I hesitated when I did answer her, but I knew to say something or she would be at the bathroom door knocking and asking me more questions. When it was time to get out of the bathtub, I really could have used some help. Instead, so that I wouldn't slip and fall, I had to get out slowly and carefully.   I didn't want anyone to see me, and I wasn't going to ask for help doing something so personal.   So I had to talk to God; all the more reason to continue asking, "Precious Lord, take my hand."

This was also the hardest moment to accept being single. A husband might have helped me with my bath and with getting dressed.   Then again, I wondered if such a suggestion would have been just one more obstacle, but since I was single, I asked God to just let me get through those moments if I had to do it alone.

I started to wonder what my life would turn into if I could never use my right arm again.   What if I could never type or walk with the movement of my arm swinging.   I was a secretary. God forbid! It was like having on an emotional cast. My instructions to exercise were to increase my arm mobility, to increase blood circulation and to strengthen the right portion of my body affected by the surgery. And—if I wanted to get better, it was about time I got started.

I tried doing my deep breathing exercises lying on my back. The deep breathing exercises were to help me relax and to expand and gently move the chest wall and lungs on the side of the surgical area. However, on my first try, I anticipated the pain so much that I couldn't relax.

Other exercises consisted of arm lifts, gripping a small rubber ball, walking my fingers up the wall, limp arm swings, and pulley and rope turning with a jump rope. Every day, I spent a portion of my day trying to do my exercises. I exercised fifteen minutes or more, gradually increasing my exercises to a full thirty minutes or more. I would get so tired and hurt so bad that I had to take a pain pill and lie down.

The pamphlets that I received from the hospital suggested that I might take a pain pill before exercising to help me relax during the exercise. Only, the medication didn't seem strong enough to last after I had finished the exercise. I would still hurt so much that when I lay down I would keep hurting as if I hadn't taken anything. Because I kept starting and stopping, I usually went over my fifteen to thirty minute time limit which probably caused much of the fatigue and after pain. I pushed myself hard, and the end result–until I realized my limits–was pain and more frustration. I knew that I needed to get back to work since my short-term disability pay wasn't enough to cover my bills.

Consequently, pretty soon I was typing every day. Looking back, I remembered genuinely hating typing in high school. The only reason that I took it in the first place was because it was a requirement, and secondly I wanted to type as well as my sister Lois. Now, I was crying and praying that I could just type again, and I kept trying until I was typing more everyday.

Shortly thereafter, I started to get through my nights and days without so much pain and frustration. Over and over, I read the booklets that I had gotten from the hospital before coming home. Everyday I would practice swinging the rope tied to a doorknob until eventually I was able to turn it over. About four weeks had passed, and although it was still difficult to walk my fingers too high up the wall, I was making pretty good progress. Likewise, I was beginning to throw and catch the little rubber jack ball.

Eventually, I could do some housework if I worked a while and sat down a while. I depended on Marfa and Lester Jr. to mow the yard. Once or twice, Lester Sr. came by to help Marfa and Lester Jr. with the mowing.

Now that Marfa and Lester Jr. had more to do, we had our frustrations about most of the work to be done inside the house too. Housework wasn't one of their fun things to do. So we finally had to sit down and have a talk about how things were going to get done. I would hear mumbling sometimes.

"It's not my time to wash dishes….," etc.

Marfa and I disagreed about almost everything that I asked her to do, and eventually she moved out with her friend. I had not expected such a battle with my children. Worst than that, I had not expected the confrontation with my ex-husband, Lester Sr. either.

One evening when Lester Sr. brought Lester Jr. home from his house, I was sitting on my living room floor talking on the telephone. Lester Sr. followed Lester Jr. inside, passing me to go to my bathroom. On his way out the front door, he came over to where I was sitting on the floor and snatched the telephone and very abruptly hung it up. Knowing that I was recovering from major surgery, the person that I was talking to thought something was wrong and called me back.

Lester Sr. took the phone, started to curse the caller and me and proceeded to say, "I run things here. You SOB. Don't you call here no more!"

By then I was on my feet and asking him to leave, but that just provoked him more. He started to slap my face until he knocked me to the floor, and every time I got up he repeatedly knocked me down again warning me of what he would do if I called the police. I kept trying to get away from him to get to the telephone. I was telling Lester Jr. to call the police, but he seemed frozen in his tracks. Then as quickly as Lester Jr. could think, he ran to his room and closed the door. Lester Sr. smelled of alcohol and cigarette smoke. Needless to say, just the fall to the floor was enough to leave me hurting, but his repeatedly knocking me around had left me hurting, more swollen and sore. I was hurting so bad, I was sure the stitches had come undone. My bandages were still on, and I was afraid that if I looked underneath I would see blood.

When Lester Sr. finally left, I called the police, and the paramedics came too. They checked me for bruises and broken bones I guess, and since they saw no blood, they saw no need to transport me to the hospital. However, when the police arrived, Lester Sr. was back at my house too. This time, he was in his other truck parked across from my house on a vacant lot. That night, he was taken by surprise when the police drove up and arrested him outside on that vacant lot. When he finally went to court, Lester Sr. received probation and remained under a restraining order for the rest of the year. For almost a year, my fears were renewed and I felt locked up in his place. Inside and out, I needed spare parts. I prayed just to think straight. I didn't feel well enough to go out and if I did, I didn't stay very long. I didn't care about a social life, and the operation gave me yet another excuse to just stay inside.

After a bitter divorce ten years prior from Lester Sr., I was forced to remember–in addition to this pain, how abusive he had been. Over a ten-year period, Lester Sr. had continued to bother me after every restraining order was over. I had to pray that I would not hate him for the things that he had already done; the drinking and drugs, the fear when the children and I already remembered when we heard his truck pull into the driveway and of all the days spent thinking, "How do I get my children and myself out. How do I leave someone like that? How do I keep my children and myself safe? When he calls my job the next time, will he really have my children and gone out of the state as he promised? What will he do? Will he kill us with his gun this time?"

I found myself, knowing all too well that I had to pray. What kind of person would deny getting help after seeing the results of the pain he had caused to a family I thought he had to have loved? How could he expose drugs and alcohol to his own son, whom he had begged God for; to a daughter that he adopted and helped raise as his own? The 37th Psalms became a daily quote. My fears were also renewed of how insecure and untrusting I would feel in future relationships for a long time—if I saw so much as a pattern of Lester Sr.'s behavior. I felt grateful that I wasn't married if this is what I would have been subjected to, and whenever I saw a couple into a loud discussion, the memory registered all too well.

By the time all of these traumas had passed, it was time to go for my chemotherapy treatments. Everything seemed so unstable all over again, and I prayed to God for strength to just get through my first hour each day and night.

Chapter 4

Starting for the Hills

_____

After my surgery, I had seen Dr. Fosmire every week at the Dallas Medical and Surgical Clinic. It was about the middle of March before I went over to the Texas Oncology Center for my first clinical appointment with Dr. Jones.

My appointment was at 2:45 p.m. that day. So at 2:05 p.m., Tom Berry dropped me off. I wished so badly that I wasn't going in by myself. I had been reluctant to consider earlier when Jerry asked me if I needed him to go with me, but sitting there, I wanted to reverse my answer.

At 2:10 p.m., I was called to the lab. I had been told that all injections, vaccinations, blood samples, and blood pressure test should be taken on the opposite side of the operative side. Clutching the little red rubber ball that I had been given for my exercises, I sat down in the chair and raised my left sleeve. The technician saw the little ball and asked where I had gotten it. She thought it was a good idea. I was squeezing it for dear life—I was so scared. After a stick to my left finger, blood samples were taken for slides. When the lab work was done, I was sent back to the waiting area to wait my time to see Dr. Jones.

While waiting for the nurse to call me, I took out my pen and started to write, hoping that I could relax.

"Every since I found out that I had cancer, everything seem upside down. My back hurts. It feels like I'm being admitted to a rest home or something. Some people look so worn and old. Their hair is either gone or almost gone, and they must be sick because it's not even gray. I wonder how many treatments they have had. I wonder if they are in pain. They walk with the aid of another person or with a cane. Either way, they appear to be in pain, and they sit so slowly and get up the same. I know I'm better than I was weeks ago—I think—but my pains and my feelings are so abstract that I can't tell the difference. I'm tired from just sitting and watching too. Well maybe I'm just scared to death."

When I put my pen and paper away, it seemed so frightening just looking around, especially not knowing what was wrong with everyone. I couldn't relax. Everybody except the clinic's staff seemed to be sick. I listened to every conversation: nurses and doctors talking to relatives of patients, nurses and doctors talking to patients, and patients talking to relatives and medical staff. I looked for clues or answers or reasons, or something—anything for comfort, to fix my mixed-up thoughts and to justify this situation.

I couldn't help but wonder what would happen if I were accidentally given too much or not enough of just one of the three drugs that were going to be administered. Or—what if I was allergic to one of the drugs and there was no other approved drug to put in its place.

"No, they don't make mistakes like that. They must have already thought about that." I thought.

Some of the patients could barely sit up straight, and I was beginning to copy their posture. I prayed for balance of my emotional and physical pain.

Thirty-five minutes passed, and I wondered if the nurses remembered that I was still there. I was the only black person there at the time, and since I didn't see more black people, I wondered if they were really going to know what to do for me. And—I know that cancer doesn't discriminate between any one race, so I had to pray just to think rationally. Seeing such severely deteriorated health around me made me feel doubtful. I put myself in their place, and I feared that I would soon know all of their pains within myself.

In an effort to keep my sanity, I tried reading magazines and brochures there on the table. I found myself reading the same thing over and over before turning to the next page, not retaining anything.

On the bright side, everyone was so kind, especially the medical staff. Then I guess that was the one sure thing they could do, and their actions came from the heart.

I looked up for a minute, and there was a blind lady—maybe in her 30's. An older lady looked across the room and smiled, "We just don't know how blessed we are." She said.

I nodded in agreement, but I knew we were blessed all right. Thank God she had someone with her. I couldn't imagine myself blind and going through chemo, and at that moment, I started to pray for that young lady. I started to concentrate on something beside my own fear. I must have prayed for everybody in that room, far away and throughout the world that day.

Finally the nurse came out and took me back to the examining room. She had me to step up on the scales to get my weight, she took my blood pressure, and she asked me a few questions. Then she gave me a little paper shirt to put on. I changed as quickly as I could, trying to relax before the nurse and Dr. Jones came back.

"What if he finds something wrong?" I thought.

I walked over to the mirror, looking to see if the scar from the surgery was ok. "How would I know anyway?" I thought.

Although there was some swelling, and I felt a little sore, there was no redness or pus that I could see. I walked back over to the examining table and sat down, taking one of the magazines to look at. I felt cold and nervous waiting.

When Dr. Jones and the nurse did come back to finish the exam, I was relieved by the things he said. Dr. Jones told me that I was doing fine, and that the treatments would not be started until my next visit. The treatments were scheduled three weeks apart, with alternate visits to see Dr. Jones and Dr. Fosmire. My blood count would be checked at the Oncology Center lab on my visits to see Dr. Jones.

When I went back to the Oncology Center for my first treatment, I wasn't any more calm than on my first visit. It's something that you don't get ready for I guess. You just walk in, sit down, and follow instructions as best you can.

When my name was called, I got up slowly as I had seen everyone else, but as fast as my weak and shaking body could. I put the magazine back on the table with the others, careful to straighten everything before moving another inch. When my name was called the second time, I raised my hand to let the therapist know that I was coming. I was moving slower than an older person.

"Please help me Lord." I thought.

When I got back to the treatment center, I felt some relief seeing some of the other patients laughing and talking while their treatment was being administered. The therapist accompanied me to the restroom where she had me wet my hair and put on a hospital cap. Afterwards, she directed me to a very comfortable leather reclining chair. Attached to the arm of the chair was a small color TV. An I.V. was waiting on the other side of that chair. Then from the refrigerator, she took another hospital cap, a cold heavy cap, and put it on my head. It felt like a block of ice.

As the therapist prepared to stick the needle in my hand, she explained the details. The three drugs to be administered were Cytoxan, Adriamycin, and Adrucil. I don't remember the order in which they were given. I was tensed at the sight of the I.V. This time, the needle was being stuck in the top portion of my hand instead of my wrist.

The therapist told me how important it was to keep still when the Adriamycin was being administered so that it wouldn't seep out of my vein and damage tissues or cause scarring. As she explained, I tried to listen and tell myself that these were the miracle drugs needed to cure my tainted cells from the cancer.

Instead, as soon as the first drug was flowing into my veins from the I.V., my attention was drawn to that moment only. I tried to concentrate on watching TV, but the cold cap was already causing my head to hurt like I had a migraine headache. Furthermore, my nose, ears, fingertips, knees and toes were feeling more numb. Like I had no more warm blood in my body, the instant coolness of the first drug chilled the rest of me. The therapist gave me a warm blanket, but seconds later were like hell on ice.

The second drug, Adriamycin—like ants in my pants, as it was explained to me by the therapist—gave me an instant site to dammed eternity. It was burning my back and my buttocks like all of the hair on my body everywhere was being consumed, leaving naked patches on my skin.

Finally, with the last drug, came the taste of a lifetime. My mental association was that of medicine in my mouth. I couldn't associate the taste with any that I had ever tasted before. Seconds later, I felt the fizz effect of a soft drink—in my nose—ready any minute, to come gushing forth through my nostrils. I felt the sensations of a sinus attack. I was sneezing, and although I wasn't trying to suppress the sneezing, it felt that way. Panic-stricken, my imagination left this world. I was so frightened that I was no longer listening to what the therapist was saying. Instead, I was then experiencing some breathing difficulty, tingling, nausea, and coolness. It was at the speed of rushing angry waters that the sensations just took charge.

"Oh, Dear God, please!" I thought.

The therapist continued to talk to me explaining and consoling, but I was so frightened that I had no positive thoughts right then. I wished someone had come with me, just to hold my hand; to know for sure that I wasn't being given too much of these drugs.

As the fizz mounted, I felt closed in and unable to move. Praying and begging God's intervention, I found myself in sympathy with the man in the Bible who was said to have been possessed with 2,000 demons.

When that first treatment was finally over, it was recommended that: I drink plenty of liquids; Watch for redness, swelling, or pain where the needle had been; Call if I experienced dizziness, fever, chills, sore throat, mouth and lip sores, wheezing, irregular heartbeat, and unusual bruising.

I was feeling too bad to go home on the bus as I had planned, so I called Lois to pick me up.   I don't remember talking very much, but when she came, I sure enough wanted to cry like the little sister her classmates once called me back in high school.

I felt that God had forgotten me big time!   I wanted to say to God—"Please, don't you ever leave me by myself to do this again.   You hear me God?   Please, just let me go on and die!"

And—as soon as those thoughts entered my mind—I knew that if it were God's intentions for me to be gone from this world, he would have taken me during my treatment.   I kept praying.   I had to pray.

I didn't feel like doing anything for myself.   I was cold, weak, nauseated and dizzy.   I was doubtful that I wanted to live—if this was what it took.   I was hungry, but I was afraid that if I ate, I would throw up.   A sip of sprite soda made my nose hurt.   It reminded me of the fizzing effects of the treatment.   Water made me feel too full.   So I just tried to sleep as much as I could.

Sure enough, I didn't eat or drink anything before sleeping, and by the next day, I had thrown up so many times. I was afraid that I was becoming dehydrated.   My stomach was sore from bending over and throwing up so much.   My throat felt dry and was hurting from nearly choking.

Lois didn't know what to get for me since she wasn't there when everything was explained. There was nothing I could think of that wouldn't make me feel sick again, regardless of what I had been told. I tried thinking of walking along the shores of clean cool waters, but I would automatically be reminded of dead fish, dirty spills, and bad smells in the air. I tried thinking of other pleasurable things like driving a brand new car, but I would think of the new smell. I tried thinking of shopping at the mall, but all I would think of were the strong smells of cologne and food. Everything reminded me of very strong odors, pain or the taste of medicine, and I felt like I was going to be sick all over again.

Desperate to feel better and determined not to call the doctor—for fear of more medicine—I started to read one of the little handbooks that was given to be at the Oncology Center, Chemotherapy, Taking Care of Yourself During Treatment by Krames Communications. It reminded me of the things my doctors had said: "While expecting some discomfort at first, go ahead and try to drink some juices and soups and eat light things like Jell-O; eat small portions; avoid foods and liquids with high acid content; try eating with plastic utensils since your mouth might feel a little sore; avoid indigestion by not eating sweets and fried foods or spicy foods, cold foods, and not drinking liquids with meals." It reminded me too, that some foods, especially red meat, would not taste the same—that it might seem too heavy to eat and swallow. It even suggested ways to relax before going to sleep such as reading, taking a walk, or talking to a friend on the phone. Only, I didn't feel like doing any of these things. I couldn't concentrate.

Even though I found all these suggestions helpful, I had waited too long to make them work. The lime Jell-O was light, easy to swallow, and left a refreshingly good taste in my mouth. However, at this point, I had to call Dr. Jones for medication to control the nausea.

Aunt Betty and one of Lois' classmates, Heneretta Jeffery, were a big help during this time for me too. They had both taken chemo some years back, and they talked to me and suggested ways of getting through the day after my treatment. They gave me tips on how to prepare my foods, and suggested that I should wear a wide brim hat or a scarf as well as long sleeves in the sun (also suggested by my doctors). They reminded me of other side effects too: hot flushes, reddish urine right after treatments, extreme hair loss that my nails would turn dark brown/purple, not to lift or carry heavy items, and to keep doing my exercises.

One day, on my way home from the doctor, I saw Heneretta. I made a comment about how really pretty her hair was, and I went on to ask her if she had a perm.

She said, "Girl, you know when I had chemo, my hair came out and it just grew back like this."

Her hair was like a newborn baby's beautiful little curly hair, and I had thought that my aunt's hair was always pretty because she went to the beauty shop.

Well, from then on, when I was going for my treatments and while I continued to recover, I talked almost every night with Heneretta and my aunt. We laughed and joked about ourselves, comparing situations and results. They made me laugh and remember that in spite of my illness, just how very blessed I was. Heneretta told me that off and on for about two years, she had taken chemo.

I knew that my aunt had been sick, but none of our family seem to have really understood what she had gone through. She said it was something that people just didn't talk about back then. She didn't have support from the family either. I felt sad for her that I hadn't been there for her. I thanked God that she and Heneretta understood my side affects and that they both knew that I wasn't just complaining-- that these were difficult times for me.

Well, time marched on, and the thought of smoke, strong odors, foods and even water still made me feel nauseated. Most of the time, I had no appetite and I slept very little at night—even after going back to work. So I usually felt very tired.

When I was feeling better, I decided to work on a book of poetry for publication. Jerry Darden came over one day while I was sitting in the cafeteria at work, and he asked me what I was writing.

"I'll let you read it, if you promise not to laugh." I said.

He promised, and we began to talk. That's when he told me that he wrote poetry too. I joked that since our birthdays were in the same month, only five days apart, that we could put together a great book.

Jerry and Thelma had been really good to me, and I wanted them to know how much I appreciated their kindness. This was it! I asked Jerry if he would like to join me in the publication of my book of poetry. We put our titles together as one. His title was INNER THOUGHTS, and mine was WHEN SHOULDERS PART. Our final decision was to use INNER THOUGHTS WHEN SHOULDERS PART. We found a publisher-Carlton Press—in a *Writer's Digest* magazine and we submitted our manuscript of poetry to them.

Jerry's writing brought more inspiration to the collection and added a lot of hope to my life. So I was very excited to have his writing going to publication with mine. He had written mostly for special occasions at his church, but his writing techniques were bold and reassuring. He appealed to young and old audiences. I, on the other hand, had always written about the things that were close to my heart. I wrote about nature's divine distributions, the love in all of us, tragedy and anything else that got my attention. I wrote to service men and their families—walking in the rain sometimes to mail the letters. It became a therapeutic measure for me.

Anyway, Jerry and I found ourselves unable to meet the financial end of our contract before Carlton Press (of nearly 100 years of business) closed its doors. So, we self-published our book. After publication, Jerry was invited to his daughter's school to read some of his poetry from the collection, and as expected, he was received well. The first critique was done by the 1993 graduating seniors at Samuel High School in Dallas, Texas.

Looking back for a moment, I remembered my mother's high hopes that I would become a successful artist one day, since I liked to draw. During my sophomore year in high school, I entered a drawing contest sponsored by the Art Instruction Schools of Minnesota, was accepted and mother signed me up for the correspondence course in commercial art. After high school, I continued to take art as my major at East Texas State University. I guess if I had been able to get to class and turn in my final project for the semester in 1971, I might have become that artist. Instead my ride didn't come that day, and it was too late to board the Continental Trailways bus in an effort to get to class. When I went to class the next day, my instructor wouldn't accept my project, and I received my very first failing grade in Art. I never went back to East Texas State University. However, that same year, I had entered a poetry contest in the English Department, and I had been awarded a dictionary in the Honorable Mention category. Following that award, I started to write more and more.

Reminiscing and trying to write in between treatments gave me some comfort. While writing about everybody's 'ups and downs,' somewhere in the middle I could see myself. Comparing, somehow, encouraged me to see my own blessings in spite of my difficulties.

After my first two treatments, I had been really sick. When I went home, I slept only two or three hours at a time, and I felt nauseated, weak, and tired most of the time. I didn't feel like eating much more than Jell-O.

Thank God I didn't have to go back to work the next day following a treatment. The treatments were always done on Fridays, and I was usually sick all weekend. Dr. Jones emphasized that I needed to stay away from people with colds and other contagious illness since I was more susceptible to infections.

With treatment number three, I asked Dr. Jones if it really was necessary to keep going. He assured me that I was at a high risk and needed to go ahead as scheduled with the other treatments. So we did, but since I had been so sick with my first two treatments, Dr. Jones suggested that I would do better to take the remaining treatments in the hospital where I would receive overnight care there also. So he admitted me to Baylor Hospital on the day of my next treatment. The surgical area was starting to heal, leaving some of the soreness behind, and because of the 'round the clock' care at the hospital I was eating better.

When I did go home, my sister-in-law came by to bring me dinner and most of the time, when she didn't, Jerry and Thelma invited me to eat with them. Lester Jr. was usually with his father and Marfa was working and with her friends.

Nonetheless, my exercises were coming along ok, and I was adjusting to the treatments until one morning when I went into the bathroom to comb my hair.

"Oh my God!" I cried.

It was like another nightmare—even though I had been told that my hair would come out. This was a big shock. My hair was coming out in my comb, chunks at a time. I saw bunches of already thinned hair, in my comb. I leaned over the sink, with both hands touching the mirror, and I just cried.

"Oh Dear God! Oh my God! Oh God please!"
I had been looking in magazines and at every woman's short hair, hoping and praying for a miracle style. I had waited to get my hair cut short—still hoping that I would have a little left in spite of what I had seen at the hospital with other patience.

My aunt's advise, "Get your hair cut real short so when it all start to come out, you'll be able to adjust emotionally."

She warned me that it would be stressful, but I had dreaded going anywhere to have my hair cut. Yet there I was in the moment. I took my scissors and whacked away until what was left of my thin little patches of hair was too short to roll over my little finger.

"I'll do something alright! I'll show you cancerous little termites just how to beat you to this thinning little mess!" I cried.

I finally decided that if I wanted to ever see the world again, I'd better go out and get a wig so I would have the courage to see it from a more positive angle. Still inside, I hated for the world to see me. I hated trying to accept all that was happening to me, and it sure was hard to adjust to the idea of wearing a wig. The top of my head was starting to feel sore.

Anyway, that day I decided, no more putting it off. I put on a little scarf, and I went to a wig shop in the shopping center just off Buckner Boulevard here in Dallas, Texas. I was glad to see that they had accessories too, but I felt embarrassed too. It felt as if everyone could see my little peel head just the way I had seen it that morning.

I bought a thick synthetic, shoulder length wig It was dark brown/black, and was hoping that my bare head didn't show through. I hated when people would walk up to me and ask if I had a perm. I hated to explain, and sometimes I didn't. I just said no, but when I simply said no, someone always wanted to feel the texture. I was so afraid that they would pull too hard or that the wind would blow it off. Other times, I heard people arguing among themselves as to whether it was real—mostly guys.

I wore a shorter curly wig too, for those times when I didn't feel like rolling or really styling my longer wig. I had hoped that after a while, people would get used to me again with shorter hair. I took more time to put on my make-up, and I wore solid clothes with special design scarves and collars to shift the attention from my hair and especially from my breast. Well, this enhanced my overall appearance all right, but it drew more attention to the total me.

One lady came up to me and said, "I almost didn't know you since you cut your hair. You look nice.

I wanted the comments to just stop. Then sometimes, I would laugh at the inside joke, "Yes, it's cut pretty short these days. Just wait until next week when the rest of it completely falls out."

All of the hair on my body was playing a disappearing act. I hoped it wasn't as evident to everyone else as it was to me, but confirmation did come. One man asked me, "Why you black women shave your legs? Do you roll that pretty hair every night?" And without letting me get a word in edgewise, "I bet you're used to guys telling you—you look good?"

I didn't feel like explaining or answering him, and I sure didn't feel like a beauty queen. So I turned and simply walked away with a smile and without much of an explanation at all. Inside, I wanted to just ask God for my old self again and for my little hair back before the wind blew that wig off or before I lost my temper the next time I was bombarded with questions like that.

Now with all of the questions and comments about my hair, hot flushes, soreness, nausea, sleepless nights, trying to be at work, and God knows what else, I became more depressed.

About my third or fourth treatment, all of my nails on my fingers and toes were turning dark brown/purple in color. My thumbs were first. I looked as if I had slammed them in a door or hit them with a hammer. They ached and my cuticles were sore. Every strand of my hair was just about gone, my mouth

was a little sore, and my appetite had to be forced. I was
starting to loose a little weight, and I felt bad, sometimes bitter.

"I feel bitterness, as I write today. It's May 29th, 1991,
and I must pray twice their once for those who say I am just
complaining. I wish that God would take this illness from this
earth once it's passed my way. I'm frustrated enough for the
entire world. Lord have mercy for their ignorance for which I
should not place blame. You have spared them the pain and
agony. They could never understand. Your cross must have
been heavier than this. I should just remember and be reminded
of the season."

I was riding the City bus to work every day, and I was
feeling really bad. The smell on the bus, the fumes on the
street, waiting on connecting buses in the sun, and literally
everything around me made me nauseated—even good smelling
perfumes and foods. Once on the bus, I was afraid that I would
throw up all over the person sitting next to me and myself.
Even the constant jolts and the motion of the bus bothered me.
I tried to remain calm, and I prayed just to make it to my stop.
Upon getting off, I prayed to get to my bathroom. Several
times, I barely cleared the steps on the bus before I was
throwing up. I always wore my tennis shoe, and I must have
washed a lot of shoe strings.

I called Jerry one evening crying, and when he answered
the phone, he asked what was wrong. I explained, "Everything
is just wrong. I'm tired Jerry. I'm tired of trying. I wish God
would just let me die if he is so good!"

Jerry listened to me talk, without interrupting. Then he
asked what he could do to make things easier for me. That's
just how Jerry is. I told him how I felt everyday, trying to ride

the bus home, and he said I could ride to work with he and Thelma.

I talked to Jerry and Orr every day, sometimes crying and determined that I was not going back to the Oncology Center for treatments ever again. They both kept telling me that I had to keep going. I was afraid that they would get tired and not listen or call anymore. I knew they couldn't understand, but to know that they were there to listen helped me more than anything else that they could have ever done.

Orr always said, "Oh you'll make it. You can't give up. What can I do?"

I explained that I knew that sometimes I said silly things, but I needed him to keep talking to me because that was how I got through my day.

Orr called everyday. He had a family member to die from cancer, so he understood some things that I was going through. We talked about growing up and times as far back in our lives as we could remember. He told me jokes, and he made me laugh. Orr always checked to see if there was something I needed. He gave me back some healing time to look and count my blessings past and present.

Jerry and Thelma called, listened and prayed with me many times—even when I didn't want to pray. They took me with them to visit with their families. They too, gave me a chance to forget about the pains. No one else heard me cry or complain so much—not even my mother. I was afraid I would worry her so much that she would have to go back to the hospital.

Mother called almost everyday, sometimes twice daily.

There were times when I didn't remember to pay my bills, no matter how much they were. When I went to the hospital for my fourth treatment, my son called to tell me that my phone and lights were off at the house. I had left money in my dresser drawer for Marfa to pay on the bills, only half the time, she wasn't even home. When I went home the money was still in the drawer. So again, I called Jerry and Thelma to ask if they would take me to pay my bills. As usual, they came.

Jerry and Thelma talked me into going to church with them one Wednesday night. When they came to pick me up, I really didn't want or feel up to going, but I went anyway.

Reverend Toney, their Pastor at Pleasant Zion Baptist Church, was in his study. Jerry asked me if I could consider talking to Pastor Toney before I made a final decision not to consider treatments.

"I guess so Jerry, but I'm still not going back. It must be my time to die," I said.

Jerry took me back to Pastor Toney's study. He had already told me that he would take me home if I didn't want to stay for all of the mid-week service, but I thought as long as I had come, I would stay.

Pastor Toney reminded me first of God's love. He explained that I couldn't give up because it wasn't myself I was giving up on. It was God; that god sees us in our darkest hour of pain.

And—Pastor Toney was going to get through to me. He was going to make me focus on life. I don't know how many times he said, "God won't put more on you than you can stand."

He talked about the struggles of Job and to give me a closer look, he talked about himself. "Baby God gave me a mission. He called me to pastor this church. I can't give up if I wanted to. You see, I get tired, but I got sense enough to know that God wouldn't put more on me than I can stand. Why should I give up if God hasn't given up? Do you see what I mean?" He said.

"Well," I said, "Reverend Toney, you just don't know how I feel and what I've been through. I don't want to take any more treatments. I'm just tired. I feel sick all the time."

Seeing that I really was loosing hope, Pastor Toney leaned forward, "Baby, if God's not ready for you to die, it won't do you any good to be tired. God's time is not out time, and all sickness is not until death. You think I didn't want to give up when I had my heart attack? Baby, that's when it's time to pray. God won't put more on you than you can stand."

Pastor Toney talked to me 30 minutes or more, and then he took my hand and prayed with me. After the prayer, he gave me a hug and said, "Sister Carter, God loves you and so do I. Don't forget that."

After that night, my niece went over to visit Ebenezer, the church where I had been a member, and she told me that Pastor Smith and the church prayed for me that morning during the alter prayer. I had not been to Ebenezer since the operation, neither had I talked with anyone at Ebenezer. I was encouraged that they thought about me, but I kept coming to Pleasant Zion because Jerry, Thelma and their daughter Glenda were always willing to pick me up.

Initially, it wasn't my intentions to join the Pleasant Zion Missionary Baptist Church, but Jerry and Thelma were so patient with me, Pastor Toney continued to counsel me, and the reception was so warm at Pleasant Zion that one Wednesday night I did join. They had come to me when I could not lift my feet to even start in any direction; when I couldn't talk about anything that was happening to me.

I had heard the choir, under the directions of Drexel Toney (Pastor Toney's son, a superb musician), and every note he played just reminded me over and over again of what Pastor Toney had said. Brother Weaver was singing, "After the Rain" (the sun will shine again), and I looked up to see this lady singing with such a joyful and sincere expression. I asked Thelma who she was, and she told me, "That's Mrs. Weaver."

"I know that's right baby!" She said, pointing her finger at her husband as he sang the lead.

Brother Weaver's base voice resounded a message of hope for all of those tomorrows that I had put aside. Then when Mary Agnew sang, "I Won't Complain," it was like a cry out from my inside—a cry to God—for strength.

That choir had filled a double prescription for me that day. I had constantly asked God for strength. I needed to stay with that church family. I wanted to sing in that choir. I needed to feel that comfort again.

It was on or about June 14th, 1991, that I was about to be admitted to Baylor for my fifth treatment. I had two more treatment to go, and I knew that I had more hills to climb. I was remembering one incident during the prior treatment that made me feel extremely nervous. When the nurse started the I.V., she had tried twice to stick the needle in the top of my hand, but she couldn't get it in my vein. I had asked her to just stop, and she called for another nurse to do the I.V.

However, on a sweeter note, with the care and watchful eye of the hospital staff, my meals were served on time, medication was given as needed, and I got plenty of rest. I had also been spared the discomfort of the cold cap. My hair, for most part, was gone by then anyway. So I guess the cold cap didn't really matter.

Growing up, I had always wanted long hair, and I was forever discouraged with my thick eyeglasses. Besides, I wondered if God listened to my requests anyway. But there's an old saying, "Be careful what you ask God for. You might just get it."

Well just when I needed an answer, God gave me one. It was months after all of my hair had fallen out. As my hair started to grow back, nothing to something—felt like really long hair. By then, I didn't care how long it was, I just wanted my hair back. I got my wish—second wish too. My eye glasses had started to feel so heavy and cool that I didn't know what was causing the pain in my face. So I went to get my eyes examined, and oh thank God for modern technology! That's when I learned that even with my prescription, I could wear contacts. I would also have to wear reading glasses with my contacts, but I had never been able to see so good in all my life!

When I went back for my follow-up visit to the Oncology Center, the next weak, I felt really good. I was better. My next treatment wasn't scheduled until on or about July 5th.

It was one of the happiest days in my life when Dr. Jones told me that I didn't have to take my last treatment if I didn't want to. I was so excited that it was over. I made flight reservations to New York, but since I had not given my daughter a graduation gift, I decided to take her with me. Unable to pay for her flight, we boarded a Continental Bus to New York, New York on August 31st. I had planned for months to go to a poetry convention there to take some of my writing.

We had a wonderful time. We spent $220 for food alone,

and our last meal in New York at the beautiful Marriott Hotel was a $20 steak burger and a soft drink—all of which we shared because I was afraid to go two blocks to McDonalds.

Upon my return, Dr. Fosmire wanted to do a biopsy on my left breast. I prayed that this was not going to be a replay. Jerry offered to go with me, and this time, I accepted. He and Thelma drove me over to the clinic that morning. Jerry stayed with me while Thelma took her mother to her doctor's appointment. When the procedure was over, there was no malignancy, and Jerry took me home. I slept some more, and I prayed some more. I didn't feel that I was going to be ok when I wasn't praying. My belief in God had gotten me through before, and God was surely my strength.

Chapter 5

God's Amazing Grace

In the shadows of God's amazing grace, the operation and five chemotherapy treatments were now history.

It felt like a mixed blessing to finally feel better again. The soreness was almost gone, and although underneath my arm felt stiff, it didn't hurt near as much. After four months, it had started to feel numb, parched maybe and hurting only when I took time to notice. However, my nails ached whenever I was in an air-conditioned room or in cool weather, and I was reminded of the cooling sensations of the cold cap. As if these recollections weren't enough, my skin tingled in warm heat, whether it was from exposure to the sun or the central heat in the room. There was a ticklish feeling underneath my skin as if my bones were moving around—just slightly out of control—just enough to cause discomfort. The hot flushed sensations were more than a flash. They seemed to last and last as if there was a needy purpose for their existence. Strong odors caused nausea still, and standing too fast caused dizziness.

It was too much, trying to keep up the yard and catch up all the utility bills. So I moved from the house to an apartment again. The apartment was nice, but there were things about that house that reminded me of just how magical life had really been.

Growing up in the country on the farm had been a life of survival, not a luxury. We were usually sick before we went to the doctor, and even then, it was only after home remedies hadn't provided relief. We only had burial insurance coverage. The amount of insurance a black man and his family could get was limited back then.

We didn't have a nightstand to place the alarm clock on beside the old iron bed; neither did we have an electric lamp to turn on in the middle of the night. Instead there was a long string which my parents tied from the ceiling light to the bed rail. In the absence of a dresser or chest, boxes held our small clothes behind a sheet hung by wire and two nails representing the corner closet. That was where our ironed clothes hang. Our shoes were kept under the beds.

We didn't have a living room. The first room of the house was also a bedroom. The tall, narrow windows were draped with tailor made curtains which my mother had sewn, using my grandmother's old sewing machine. When company came, they sat on the porch or we brought the chairs and the wooden bench from the kitchen table for them to sit in. There was no soft cushion to put in the seat of the chairs or on the bench. Sometimes, company sat on the edge of the bed—a carefully made bed in the front room—where the good bedspread was a cover. Mother used the cloth sack that baking flour came in to make designed pillowcases for our feather and cotton filled pillows.

Saturday nights and after church on Sunday evenings, we visited daddy's brothers in Wolf City or mother's mother in Greenville to watch television. Since there was no telephone or TV in our house until after the sixties, we all learned at an early age to improvise. My grandfather (mother's father) lived with us for a while, and although I was somewhat of a shy child in public, I loved to make him laugh. Since he was blind, he was the perfect audience.

Even when we all gathered around the radio to listen, it was always a family affair. It was like watching TV to listen to Lone Ranger, Amos and Andy, and Gunsmoke. Besides the gospel singing on radio station KNOK, we listened to records that mother and daddy ordered from Nashville, Tennessee. I remember such recording artist as the Staple Singers (daddy's favorite), Mahalia Jackson (My mother's favorite), Reverend C.L. Franklin, and Aretha Franklin's songs, "Precious Lord" and "Never Grow Old" (my favorites). When the KNOK station in and around the Dallas area (in Texas) didn't come in clear, we sometimes listened to local stations which played mostly country, blues and jazz. We were privileged to hear recording artist Johnny Cash, Diana Shore, Fats Domino, B.B. King, Chuck Berry, Nat King Cole, James Brown, Little Richard, and Ella Fitzgerald—to name a few.

My parents knew what we were capable of from observation. They knew what was going on at our schools too because they came to school functions. They were not surprised at what we could do because they rehearsed with us at home. They knew the songs that we sang because they taught us and sang most of them with us.

The radio was in their room—the entertainment center of the house. We listened, joked and played together. Radio was a luxury, and we didn't dare turn the station when mother and daddy were gone or out of the room either. It was treated with the same emphasis as the family car.

We had regular toys I guess—for the times: white dolls, paper dolls, colors and coloring books, jack and ball sets. It was rare to get a black doll if there were very many on the market back then. I wish I could say that I even saw a black doll. Sometimes we would cut a model from the sears catalogue and then find the clothes in the same catalogue and cut them out to fit the model that we had cut out of that same catalogue. My sister, my brother and I played connect the dot on paper with mother and daddy, but, we all had our unique interest wherein we could just have quiet time to ourselves. I had a paint set, my brother had a wagon, and my sister had a bicycle. Mother had her sewing and daddy had his garden and home brewery.

When my father and brother died in 1961, we lived in a little community called, "Jot 'M' Down, Texas. We had never lived anywhere long enough to get used to it. When the crops were done, it was almost always time to move on to another town. We usually lived just outside town—in the country, so Jot 'M' Down was a town to me since people actually lived next door. Our neighbors had always been miles down the road from us. I don't know how mother and daddy managed back then, except that God surely had to have been a part of their plans.

In 1961, daddy died in his brother's living room of a heart attack. When my sister Lois, my youngest brother Melvin and I came home from school, they told us that daddy had died.

72

I didn't believe them at first. In my mind, I wondered why God would take him from us.

I was hurting inside with so many questions that I needed God to answer: "Who will drive us to church on Sundays? Who will take us to watch TV on Saturday nights at Uncle Will's house? Oh God, how am I supposed to grow up without my daddy to help my mother anyway?"

I just thought that they had to be teasing. I was afraid for my daddy to be closed up in that coffin without us. When he came home, he would ask my mother where we were. I was so afraid that I was about to cry, and I didn't want to. I was so upset with God. I thought I had to talk to God a lot to get him to understand that I wasn't ready to die, in spite of the fact that our family had always gone everywhere together.

For the funeral, daddy's children from his first marriage came, and we all saw each other for the first time. We were excited about seeing them. I felt good knowing that we had other brothers and another sister: Alvin Jr., Eddie, J.D. and Clarine. I remember thinking how really pretty Clarine was, how tall she was, but mostly how she must have missed daddy too. I couldn't imagine being without him.

Little did we all know that in several months, our youngest brother would also die? He was ~~eight~~ ten years old, and that was especially hard for me. He had drowned in the little pond back of the house we lived in. We played together all the time. And—again, I asked God why he had to take my brother. Would my daddy be able to keep my little brother from being scared in his grave?

"I sure prayed, Lord I hope so."

This kept getting more confusing to me. I was afraid to sleep in that house anymore.

"Lord, please don't come get me too," I prayed.

Again, I prayed to just be all right—I guess to understand.

Anyway, my mother was no sharecropper—thank God. It must have just been time to leave there. We moved to Greenville, Texas, where she bought a house with what insurance money she had left over (a down payment of $200). It needed repairs everywhere, but that old house was ours. The neighborhood was clean; with people who cared about each other. The house note was $25 a month. Mr. Grundy, the owner of Grundy's Funeral Home (in Greenville, Texas) had helped mother relocate and get the property on Marshall Street.

I remember thinking, "Mr. Grundy must be the richest black man that I had seen yet."

He drove the shiniest, big black car. I didn't know, at the time, that it was one of the family cars used in the funerals.

Mr. Grundy died before any repairs could be done to fix up the house. The roof leaked so bad in the back room that nothing of great value was kept back there; mostly clothes in boxes that lay on an old iron bed. A large piece of thick plastic was always spreaded over the bed and the boxes so that the rain and dust wouldn't ruin everything. I would go back there and sing sometimes because of the insulated sound.

That was a fun room, and probably could have been fixed up to be a nice room for my mother's bedroom. Instead, she slept in a little twin size bed in the corner of the living room, the first room in the house. I prayed that one day I would earn enough money to buy my mother a new house.

The other bedroom was the room that my sister and I shared. The wall paper was peeling, and the base structure of the wall was exposed. Mother had some plasterboard (sheetrock) put up, but we never had enough money to get the room painted or to get more wall paper.

The bathroom was in need of repairs even worst. I had tried fixing the floor. The floor became a see-through window to the ground underneath the house. A piece of linoleum was kept over it. The wet wood underneath the linoleum would buckle and snails would come crawling up through the bathroom floor, lingering around the plumbing and corners of the bathroom. We would melt them away with table salt. That seemed so nasty. So I was always trying to help keep the floor covered with linoleum, and nailing down the rain buckled wood until it rotted so bad from the rain leaking inside.

The kitchen was starting to need repairs too. The counter tops were in such bad shape, I bought some topping and nailed it on myself. The back kitchen door, leading outside, could have used some weather stripping, but mother used what she had, usually a towel or quilt to keep the cold out and the heat in.

The yard, on the other hand, was big and pretty as any of the others in the neighborhood. Looking at our house from the outside, there was no way to tell that it was in such bad shape on the inside. I helped with the yard, and pretty soon, I learned how to trim the hedges, dig weeds out of the flower beds, mow the lawn and edge with mother's sewing scissors.

Mother worked as a maid for Dr. and Mrs. Cantrell, at fifty cents an hour, four to twelve hours a day—more or less. Almost always she walked to work in shoes that had no business knowing cold weather. She never got drivers license to drive daddy's old car before she had to sell it. The Cantrells would bring her home when it was dark sometime. They picked me up to baby sit their two children in mother's place when they were going out.

It didn't matter what her work schedule was, when mother was home, she still found time to read and sing with my sister Lois and me. Mother was dramatic in her story telling. When she got to a word that she couldn't pronounce, when would spell it out-loud for us, and sometime we would all get tickle.

We always had magazines, the Texas almanac, reference books, Children's Bible storybooks, and a large family Bible. She read almost every night to us from the Children's Bible storybook until we were thirteen and fourteen. We would practice from the Baptist Hymnal and other gospel songbooks together (since we were all in the church choir at New Jerusalem Missionary Baptist Church). One of the songs that we often sang together was "In the Garden."

Years later, after my sister and I had moved away, while mother and my little nephew slept, the house caught on fire. They got out of the house safely, but the structure burned to the ground. That's when mother bought another house.

Consequently, keeping with family tradition, I accumulated a variety of reading materials on numerous subjects for my children. Included was a large family Bible—with references—and on the same shelf, several supplemental Biblical textbooks; how to kinds of instruction books (that I used to enhance my own job skills since dripping out of school at East Texas State University); other specialty kinds of books (poetry, interior decorating, art, sewing, architecture, music, children's story books, magazines, dictionaries—in English, Spanish, French and Sports) and other cultural books.

The fireplace, though more elaborate than the old wood burning stove—in the middle of the room where I grew up with my mother and father—was still symbolic in its representation of the same warmth and memories of family. Upon the mantle were pictures of my parents and my youngest brother—taken in the mid-fifties—along with baby pictures of my children from the early seventies, an anniversary clock that my son bought for me one Christmas, and a little gold tone trophy that he had been awarded at his school. Marfa had gotten a trophy for her achievements in basketball, and for several years, Lester Jr. had wanted one too. So when he finally earned one of his own, we put it on the mantle.

A green sofa, with a touch of peach and white was in front of a bay window, where sheer store bought curtains hang over white mini blinds. New beginnings were in that living room. The mantle was trimmed with a glossy white coat of paint opposite the white satin textured walls.

I had memories of that same fresh air in the house where I grew up. Back then, every room had it's own air conditioner—if there was a window to raise, and it was occasionally shared with lady bugs and mosquitoes. Now, looking around me, I felt the blessed wonders of central air and heat, and ceiling fans with optional three speeds to circulate the air and heat without having to raise a single window. The white vaulted ceiling complemented clean white walls that made my life richer than any amount of money ever could.

It had not been until the early eighties that my mother's house entertained such amenities as carpet and ceiling fans—even with the second house that she bought. Pieces of old rug or carpet parts had been the protection of our bare feet from the splintered, hardwood floors and cool winter months.

I remember some very difficult times in our house when we needed things that we sill couldn't afford, but I was reminded—even then—that God gave us people to help. Besides our family, the neighbors, church members, and teachers—but always church members and teachers. We were active in the church. Mrs. Morris, our pastor's wife, took me with her and their daughter Donna almost everywhere they went. Mother didn't have the resources to do some of the things with me that she would liked to have done, but she allowed me to be in the company of others who could offer good directions.

I was always trying to be creative, while being content, even when all was not the best. I remember having a pair of blue penny loafers. These shoes must have been a touch of class to me. On Sundays, I polished them black and on Mondays, I washed that black polish off and wore those blue penny loafers to school. Mrs. Morris noticed that I needed some shoes, and she bought me some.

I had a job at one of the elementary schools cleaning up that paid $25.00 a month, and I would baby sit Donna for Reverend and Mrs. Morris, and anybody else when I could. I drew pictures and typed for people too. My sister would sew simply slip-on dresses for people.

Being a teenager seemed to have required using what I had in creative as well as responsible ways. Now, as an adult, I'm a witness that God will not only reward you in heaven, but he will reward us with things we need right here on earth. It was a challenge for me in my life, but God used his resources to work his miracles.

The choir at Pleasant Zion sang a song "I'm A Testimony, Just Look At Me!" Pastor Toney said, "Don't leave the church—don't leave the fellowship of God. He won't force you to come back, but he'll stand patiently waiting. There is nowhere to go. Just look at what happened to the prodigal son. There is no better place to go. Have confidence and wait."

Thank God I had some tried and true family values to lean on, fellowship with God, and Christian people willing to carry out his will. As I looked around the room, it brought me back in focus with the distance that I have traveled. It was like God had granted me a fairy tale.

My children and I have witnessed many scars, but we have witnessed far more blessings. So finally, I understood dying. I had been dying a little after all of these experiences. I now understand God's eternal goodness even more; his amazing grace.

He looked beyond my faults and supplied all of my needs. To this day, even though some of the side affects still slow my day, I'm able to go on with my daily task. The hot flushes still come without warning. My skin still tingles in warmth and is chilled (especially my nails) in cool environments. Strong odors, occasionally still causes nausea, and there are some foods that I don't care for. Cigarette smoke—just the thought—makes me feel sick. Sweets are no longer a controlling factor in my diet. Soft drinks sometime make me feel nauseated too, but the wheels of faith are still turning—thanks to Good's amazing grace.

May this book serve as a brand new reflection of faith; a renewal for all who have doubts of God's goodness and mercy, and as a message of thanks to all who were so kind and obedient to God's will for my sake.

A Note from the Author.........

It was a reminder of God's special love writing this book;
an encouraging step out again to new and positive
directions.

"For I reckon that the sufferings of this present time are not worthy to be compared with the glory which shall be revealed in us."

Romans 8:18

Take care of yourself.